Healthcare

Marketing, Sales, *and* Service

Healthcare

Marketing, Sales, and Service

AN EXECUTIVE COMPANION

John F. O'Malley

ACHE Management Series
Health Administration Press, Chicago, Illinois

05 04 03 02 01   5 4 3 2 1

Library of Congress Cataloging-in-Publication Data

O'Malley, John F.
   Healthcare marketing, sales, and service : an executive companion / by John F. O'Malley.
      p. cm.
Includes bibliographical references and index.
ISBN 1-56793-150-2
    1. Medical care—United States—Marketing.   2. Health maintenance organizations—United States—Marketing.   I. Title.
RA410.56.O46   2000
362.1'068'8—dc21   00-047292
                                            CIP

The paper used in this publication meets the minimum requirements of American National Standard for Information Sciences—Permanence of Paper for Printed Library Materials, ANSI Z39.48-1984. ∞ ™

Health Administration Press
A division of the Foundation of the
   American College of Healthcare Executives
One North Franklin Street, Suite 1700
Chicago, IL 60606–3491
(312) 424–2800

Contents

Preface

AFTER MANY YEARS of conducting 60 to 70 national healthcare marketing, sales, and customer service seminars annually, I realized the need for a strategic guide for healthcare executives — a quick read that deals with strategic allocation and stresses the importance of marketing, sales, and service.

I understand that most healthcare executives are striving to remain viable within strategic reimbursement, operational, and clinical quagmires. They are seldom able to surface long enough to heed the market's call for change. Herein lies the problem. A healthcare entity cannot succeed by cutting costs alone. For decades, we pillaged the geese that laid golden reimbursement eggs, using creative financing, bundling, *un*bundling, and cost shifting. The geese are finally meeting their end on managed care's chopping block. As an industry, we have to migrate to a better healthcare delivery and reimbursement system. We must realize that long-term fixes will only evolve through trial and error. We must lead by influence, not position.

Peter F. Drucker (1985), world-renowned business guru, said: "Finance is not the center of the business universe, marketing is. And because its purpose is to create a customer, the business enterprise has two, and only two, basic functions: marketing and innovation. Marketing and innovation produce results (customers). All the rest are costs!"

A healthcare entity that operates based solely on reimbursement will run into trouble down the road. Our current financial management of healthcare, based on reimbursement options, is a testimonial to that end. Some healthcare executives have slid into reimbursement's tar pit, struggling to free themselves while slowly sinking deeper and deeper into uncertainty. To be free from the pitfalls of healthcare means to strategically grow your business from a profitable base without compromising patient care. It also means being able to create and manage change, which in turn requires a clear mission, core values, and the ability to work outside the status quo.

In this book, I try to encourage readers to free themselves from the box of the status quo. As Albert Einstein once said, "You can't solve current problems with current thinking. Current problems are the result of current thinking."

My resources stem from more than 25 years of personal experience; a mountain of books, articles, and publications, and from the ideas of others smarter than I am. I've learned to put "care-ism" before capitalism in all my thoughts, and I constantly remind myself that what humanity yearns for is an ideal life in a pragmatic world.

Because healthcare is a numbers game—requiring the right payer mix, reimbursement mix, patient mix, clinical mix, and the right managed care plan—many executives focus on the daily numbers. In doing so, they overlook the fact that numbers can be misleading, and forget the major effect that marketing, sales, and service can have on their organization's long-term success.

The purpose of this book is to reengineer the healthcare executive's mindset about the holy triad of business growth: marketing, sales, and service. The book intends to help healthcare executives enhance their ability to lead through changing and challenging times. Things have to change to remain the same. In other words, if you are number one today, you must change to be number one tomorrow.

This book is divided into three parts, covering marketing, sales, and service. Section One, Marketing, deals with the key principles, methodologies, and strategies that affect those who control the referral source and, therefore, the delivery of healthcare.

Section Two, Sales, covers important selling methods and management tools. It stresses that those who help others to succeed will succeed themselves.

Section Three, Service, unlocks the mystery to gaining ultimate employee and customer satisfaction. Those who can coach their organization to change for the better can gain the most loyal customers.

The contents of this book can be summed up by saying that marketing, sales, and service are critical to all healthcare providers' long-term success. I hope that this book can help healthcare executives lead their organizations to thrive in today's competitive climate and exploit tomorrow's new challenges.

*This book is dedicated to David Ross O'Malley,
my beloved brother and best friend, who went
on to glory May 7, 2000.*

SECTION ONE

Marketing

What Is Marketing?

THIS CHAPTER PRESENTS a bird's-eye view of marketing. It characterizes the overriding purpose of marketing and the core characteristics of successful healthcare marketing. In addition, it suggests the psychology behind customer perception and behavior as a basis for marketing strategy and tactics. Later chapters will address more specific marketing activities such as branding, Internet marketing, and referral databases.

Every marketing guru and university professor has his or her own definition of marketing. Simply stated, marketing is a battle for a person's mind. It employs the art and science of identifying and understanding people's perceptions, interests, and desires. Marketing monitors why, how, and when people satisfy their perceptions, interests, and desires and attempts to influence the decision process. Marketing also plans and executes the conception, pricing, promotion, and distribution of ideas, goods, and services. The goal is to create internal and external exchanges that satisfy individuals and organizations. Marketing is all about people, just like business and healthcare are about people. Successful marketing is built on strategic human bonds. Personal relationships occur before business relationships.

Not only does marketing drive an organization's competitive position and overall success, marketing activities influence a broad range of activities and people within a healthcare organization, from planning to the medical staff.

AREAS INFLUENCED BY MARKETING

Public relations	Community relations
Customer service	Community health assessment
Referral acquisition	Advertising/promotions
Referral source relations	Direct mail/newsletters
Medical staff	Consumer-direct marketing
Nonmedical staff	New business acquisition
Nonphysicians	Business development
Strategic planning	Business-to-business marketing
Sales management	Business coalition relationship
Managed care plans	Product line management
Patient satisfaction	Product and service branding
Employee satisfaction	Crisis management
Consumer research	Development fund support
Government relations	

Marketing requires common sense and, especially in today's competitive marketplace, a commitment to success not unlike the commitment necessary in warfare. Hence, marketing's two best strategies are:

1. do not waste time and money; and
2. create an influential presence that drives your competition to self-destruction while you succeed.

LEADERSHIP AND MARKETING

Marketing is not that difficult when you understand its essence. As a healthcare executive, you should be focusing on leadership; establishing the organization's mission, vision, and values; and communicating in a way that creates bonds. Monitor the rest with an inquisitive mind, an observant eye, and a receptive ear.

The following paragraphs offer an overview of the leadership activities that pave the way for successful marketing.

Executive Leadership

Marketing does not stand a chance of succeeding without executive understanding and support. Executives must have a vision for the organization, and marketing helps them see farther, broader, sooner, and with more insight than the competition. Remember the insightful words of Peter Drucker (1985), "Finance, is *not* the center of the business universe, marketing is."

Informed Staff

Every employee needs to know the executive's vision. Proper communication between executive management and employees will produce mutual ownership, expected change, and desired performance.

Vision, Mission, and Values

The larger the organization, the more critical it is to have a statement of vision (future), mission (guidance), and values (ethics). Vision, mission, and values set the organization's focus. Your vision statement tells employees where you want to go. Your mission statement informs them how you expect to get there.

And your value statement conveys how you are going to treat employees and customers along the way.

Planning

Next comes the business plan (where you want to go), the financial plan (how to sustain the journey), and the marketing plan (how you are going to get there). But never engage in these plans without your vision, mission, and values. Remember marketing strategy number one: "Do not waste time and money." Creating plans without your vision, mission, and values is a waste of time, and time is money.

Marketing Strategy

Marketing is the critical arm of strategic planning. You only have three core strategies from which to choose:

1. Proactive: Leadership-oriented dominance marketing
2. Reactive: Catch-up-oriented response marketing
3. Nonactive: Extinction-oriented status quo marketing

For example, a nonactive strategy regarding medical errors results in a reactive strategy to address the abuse. However, a proactive strategy would resolve abuses before they occur. The healthcare industry has the choice of changing proactively on its own initiative or responding reactively to dissatisfied patients and watchdog agencies. Proactive marketing is the only winning strategy.

Internal Marketing

An organization's internal marketing deals with three areas that affect the delivery of your products and services: 1) the service environment, 2) employee satisfaction, and 3) customer satisfaction. No matter their positions within an organization, all employees are in marketing and sales and need a statement to that effect in their job descriptions.

External Marketing

External marketing includes the traditional marketing functions such as research, advertising, and public relations. In addition to these vehicles, healthcare marketing grows the business by the acquisition, retention, and cultivation of referral sources, patients, and managed care plans.

Bonding

Always remember that human bonding comes before business bonding. The best way to promote human bonding in healthcare is by ensuring that your customers perceive compassion, not greed.

ESSENTIAL ACTIVITIES OF MARKETING

Now we will explore the specific focus of marketing activities. Marketing majors have long been taught the four Ps of marketing: product, price, place, and promotion. Healthcare marketing, however, has ten Ps, as briefly described below. Subsequent chapters of this book will cover these key elements of marketing in more detail.

People

Employees are the most important element in any healthcare organization. They must be knowledgeable, creative, confident, and willing to exercise sound business and clinical judgment.

Products

Services are also included with products. They must be appealing to existing and future referral sources, patients, and payers. They must establish a unique image and delivery approach, while achieving maximum medical outcomes in the face of competition.

Profitability

All services provided need to be profitable in nature. No profit, no mission. In time, break-even business will break your heart and kill your organization.

Productivity

Maximize time, labor, and capital to help your organization and customers profit.

Points

Service access points—hospitals, clinics, and offices—are vital to delivering one's products and services. They must be easily available to referral sources and their patients.

Pricing

Provide attractive pricing. You, as the healthcare provider, will profit when you offer value pricing to the payer, referral source, and patients.

Promotion

Educate payers, plans, physicians, referral sources, and patients. Promote your organization with action-generating advertising, newsworthy public relations, and community healthcare events.

Patients

Trust is the foundation of patient satisfaction and loyalty. And patients, not shareholders, should be the foundation of your organization.

Perception

Perception is reality. Your target audience's perception of you and your organization determines its willingness to give you its business.

Proactivity

Today's status quo leaders become tomorrow's followers. You must make a commitment to action to win customers. Where contentment resides, progress is never invited.

PSYCHOLOGY AND MARKETING

One aspect of human relationships that is key to marketing is understanding the psychology of your customers. Once you understand how your customers and prospective customers think, introducing them to your products and services becomes easier. This psychology is manifested in the various stages a consumer goes through as he or she first encounters your organization and then begins to experience its services (see Table 1.1.). If through your marketing, communication, and customer service you are able to take a consumer through these stages successfully, you will have a customer who actually markets *for* you through what is known as loyalty referring. The psychology behind loyalty referring can fine-tune your approach to marketing, advertising, promotions, selling, and customer service.

TABLE 1 1　PSYCHOLOGY BEHIND LOYALTY REFERRING

Stage	Thought Pattern	Action
Preoccupation	I cannot recall hearing about you	None
Awareness (prospect)	I heard about you	Indifference
Knowledge	I know who you are	Building a familiarity with you
Perception	I know what you embody	Forming an opinion about you
Desire (qualified prospect)	I want to refer to you	Seeking you out
Experimentation (referral source)	I will try your services	Validating your quality and claims
Fortification	Did I make the right choice about you?	Reinforcing personal beliefs about you
Satisfaction	I like you and your services	Feeling good about you
Promotion	I will tell others about you	Transferring personal beliefs about you to family and peers
Repeat (loyal referrer)	I want to refer to you again	Reliving the good feeling you provided

Psychology also plays an important role in the specific strategies and tactics you employ in marketing. Marketing must address how people make purchasing decisions and how they respond to various kinds of communication and information. The following points will help you evaluate or create marketing strategies, approaches, and activities.

- The buying *it* (tangible) and the buying *in* (conceptual) decisions are made subconsciously.
- You reach a prospect's subconscious by repetition. Deliver a short message repeatedly. An advertisement is run a minimum of six times before it reaches the target's mind.
- Left-brained people (typically right handed), about 85 percent of the population, respond best to marketing and selling approaches that provide sequential and logical information.
- Right-brained people (typically left handed), about 15 percent of the population, respond best to marketing and selling approaches that are striking, abstract, and aesthetic.
- Great marketing and selling communications combine both emotion and logic. Lead with emotion, follow with logic.
- Successful businesses bond with their customers on both a human level and a business level. The stronger the human bond, the greater the business bond.
- All marketing and selling approaches deliver a stated message compounded with an interpreted message. The stated message is *what* you say. The interpreted message is *how* you say it. Interpreted messages are usually the stronger of the two. Great marketing and selling approaches focus on the total message.
- Common approaches to marketing and selling both change a prospect's attitude and modify a prospect's behavior. Great marketing and selling approaches aim to shape attitudes

while exposing prospects to a high frequency of "act-now" opportunities.

- Prospects are not always comfortable buying new products or services. Great marketing and selling approaches put prospects at ease with free information, consultation, trial periods, demonstrations, and samples.
- Full-color marketing and selling materials increase data retention and the tendency to buy. Research shows that color suggests quality. Great marketing and selling approaches exploit the use of color, including colorful actions and colorful speech.
- Prospects will look more favorably toward you and your organization if they perceive that you put their well-being before your own. Great marketing and selling approaches put care-ism before capitalism.
- Prospects like to feel special. Great marketing and selling efforts customize products and services to each individual prospect.

ACHIEVING MARKETING GOALS

The remaining sections in this chapter address several of the core goals of marketing and offer succinct strategies for gaining patient share, marketing new products, and differentiating your products.

Gaining Patient Share

When attempting to gain your desired patient (market) share of a product line or service, consider using the following 14 steps as a guide.

1. Delineate your service area. What are the geographical boundaries?

2. Determine potential consumer interest in and need for your products and services.
3. Determine the decision makers who need your products and services.
4. Develop your ideal customer/consumer profile. Your best customers consistently provide the highest profit and volume (loyalty).
5. Analyze your service area's demographic and socioeconomic data.
6. Determine consumption trends for your products and services.
7. Determine potential customer/consumer interest levels for your products and services.
8. Conduct a benefit-to-change analysis based on saving the customer/patient time and money.
9. Determine your desired primary and secondary consumer/patient by considering reimbursement, procedure, and profitability.
10. Determine your reimbursement mix for each product line and service.
11. Determine the actual cost to deliver your products and services. Research activity-based costing (ABC) to get the jump on cost assessment.
12. Conduct a cost-to-continue analysis. Learn what it costs your customers to be loyal.
13. Conduct a competitive response analysis and create a proactive counter strategy.
14. Create a marketing action plan that achieves your vision and business goals. Such a plan needs to include management of the following elements:
    - Budget creation
    - Advertising and promotion
    - Referral acquisition, retention, and cultivation
    - Product development and delivery

- Research and database
- Customer service and patient satisfaction
- Competitive intelligence gathering

When considering this plan, you must also consider who will manage the process.

Marketing New Products

According to a 1994 best-in-class study jointly conducted by the Boston Consulting Group, the Management Roundtable, and Product Development Consulting, researchers found that of 550 manufacturers, the most successful product innovators involved their marketing staff in development and their engineering staff in marketing. And when looking at sources of new product ideas, engineers and marketers seemed to contribute more than senior management. The same holds true for healthcare organizations. Physicians and nurses are your clinical "engineers" and should collaborate with your marketing people to contribute to your success. Do not base your products and services on reimbursement alone.

Differentiating Your Products and Services

You must actively differentiate your products and services from the competition. Your customers and patients must perceive a significant advantage in dealing with you over your competition. Differentiating your products and services successfully becomes easier by using the following strategies.

- Establish a higher product-quality perception in the mind of your customers and end users.
- Consistently deliver superior customer service and patient satisfaction.

- Excel in the marketplace by exceeding customer expectations.
- Create professional and informal relationships that foster long-term customer loyalty.
- Enable business technology to maximize communications between you and your customers.
- Use information technology to maximize data collection and analysis.
- Employ evidence-based medical technology and procedures to maximize your patients' outcomes.
- Create realistic policies and procedures that make doing business with you easier for your customers and patients.
- Focus on speed, security, and safety—three of the driving forces in the future of healthcare.
- Think retail, not healthcare, in delivering your product and service.

SUMMARY: THE SEVEN SECRETS TO PROVIDER SUCCESS

A successful provider always focuses on delivering what customers want and on achieving a maximum medical outcome with minimal technical expertise, in the shortest time, and at the lowest cost. The tenets of marketing and customer service can be summarized into the following seven secrets of provider success.

1. Offer attractive pricing (lowest cost-to-outcome ratio).
2. Deliver the best customer service and ultimate patient satisfaction (internal and external).
3. Deliver accepted quality (benchmark your core service).
4. Employ competitive-edge information technology (faster and more accurate, with less labor).
5. Practice evidence-based medicine (best-practice mentality).
6. Demonstrate care-ism before capitalism.

7. Keep promises within your services and delivery system (walk the walk that others only talk).

Healthcare providers are rapidly discovering that having a high-quality product or service means little if that product or service is "me-too" driven — that is, perceived by customers as similar to what the competition provides. The customer's perception is the true barometer of success.

MOVING AHEAD

With this overview of the concepts and key concerns of healthcare marketing, we can move ahead to some more specific activities involved in establishing and carrying out a marketing plan. One of this book's core tenets is that organizations that offer similar services are often perceived as "me-too" providers. The next chapter provides strategies and tactics that will help you distinguish your products and services from the competition.

2
Conquering the "Me-Too" Syndrome

PERHAPS THE MOST important goal of marketing is distinguishing yourself from your competitors. Like most industries, healthcare has many me-too providers—the passive followers. If one creates a new product, others quickly follow, and their copycat efforts can eventually convert the originator into a me-too provider. The chances are good that your organization is a me-too provider if your products and services are also offered by others. For example, if I have a nagging sore throat and Dr. Peters is the only physician in town treating sore throats, she has a captive customer base. However, if other area doctors treat sore throats, Dr. Peters offers a me-too service. You may believe that your products and services are better than the competition's, but the competition believes that its products and services are better than yours.

Consider the example of computer tomography (CT) scanning. In 1972 when EMI introduced their computer tomography

17

brain scanner to the medical community, they had the only CT system in the world. Hence, EMI had an exclusive, or captive, market: If you wanted a CT brain scanner, you had to do business with EMI. Without even trying, EMI branded its CT technology. Everyone referred to a CT scan as an EMI. No copycat manufacturer existed, though many were getting ready to pounce on the lucrative market. Today, many me-too manufacturers offer CT scanners, but where is EMI?

This chapter offers a variety of strategies and techniques for conquering the me-too syndrome—providing products and services that stand out and letting your stakeholders know that you are a distinct and superior provider.

SEPARATION STRATEGIES

The following separation strategies will help you distinguish yourself from the me-too horde.

Save Your Customers Time and Money

Or better yet, *make* them money. Analyze every customer activity to figure out how much time and money you save them. Take a new perspective on what you do and how you benefit your customers. Position your company priorities and infrastructure for tomorrow's opportunities. Table 2.1 gives many examples of how you can save your customers time and money.

Find New Ways to Do Old Things

Do them faster, more accurately, and with less labor. Look at an activity and decide how it can be done better using enabling technology. As an example, assume you receive $100 reimbursement per patient and treat three patients in a given period to gross $300. Now assume that new reimbursement regulation reduces the

TABLE 2.1.   SAVING CUSTOMERS TIME AND MONEY

Patients	Referral Sources	Employers	Family Members	Vendors
MMOMT/MC*	Accurate testing	MMOMT/MC	Hassle-free access	Access
Accurate testing	Assistance	Quick return to work	Convenience	Education
Assistance	Caring	Cost effective	Visitor service	Communications
Caring	Charges	Customer service	Patient satisfaction	Compliance
Charges	Communications	Communications	Caring	
Communications	Compliance checking	Employee satisfaction	Assistance	
Compliance checking	Convenience		Communications	
Convenience	Customer service		Education	
Customer service education	Education		Off-hour hotline	
First-time accuracy	First-time accuracy		Quick referral	
Long-term satisfaction	Managed care plans			
Medical expertise	Medical expertise			
Off-hour hotline	Off-hour hot line			
Quick access	Patient satisfaction			
Quick referral	Report usability			
Transportation	Quick access			
	Quick referral			
	Scheduling			
	Transportation			

* MMOMT/MC = Maximum Medical Outcome at Minimal Time and Minimal Costs

$100 to $50. In order to retain the $300 gross revenue, you must either double the number of patients seen in the same period or halve the time spent on treating patients. In both scenarios, whatever you did before must now be done faster. Increasing the speed of an activity typically increases the chances for errors while doing it. Enabling technology needs both increased speed and accuracy. A third option to regain the $300 in revenue is to reduce your operating costs. Enabling technology must also reduce activity labor, which may lead to eliminating staff positions.

Focus on the Delivery System

Think retail, not healthcare. Healthcare and medical intervention are services, so start thinking like a retailer. How can you best allow customers to make contact with your system? How can you best guide customers through the delivery system? How can you streamline your system so that it is less complex and more logically organized from the customer's point of view?

Rethink All Processes

Always keep pace with your customers' interests, and turn those interests into products and services. Dance with your customers, and let your customers lead. Be creative, progressive, and proactive; success is born of innovation, not imitation.

THINK RETAIL, NOT HEALTHCARE

The true secret to marketing healthcare services is to think in terms of retail. Ask yourself, how would Neiman Marcus run a hospital? How would Nordstrom operate a skilled nursing facility? How would Tiffany & Company serve customers of a home care agency? These companies all share three things: top-line service, quality products, and higher-than-average prices.

To begin the path toward emulating the customer service of top retailers, consider the following strategies.

Enhance Customer Encounters

The little things count the most. Enhance the everyday things that customers encounter, such as places, people, and procedures.

Enhance Information Exchanges

Make it easy for prospects and customers to give information to you and get information from you. Train your customer service operations in telephone etiquette. Disconnect protocols and build up your web site.

Enhance Related Product Encounters

Determine relationships among products and services. Cross-educate and cross-sell. Convert the patient room television into an audiovisual billboard where patients can also take a virtual tour of your offerings (for example, the rehabilitation center).

Enhance Growth Around Core Business

Hospitals have gotten into every conceivable healthcare business. Some are even in the insurance business and wondering why their HMO is more of an anchor than a lifesaver. Buying physicians' practices is also weighing them down. Consider the Pepsi Cola company. It excels at producing and marketing flavored colored water. Pepsi once expanded into the fast-food industry as a short-cut to selling its core product by acquiring Pizza Hut, Kentucky Fried Chicken, and Taco Bell. The gross margins associated with selling colored water were great; the fast-food industry's gross margins, however, were not. Stock value went down and shareholders got upset. Pepsi quickly refocused on its core business and sold its fast-food restaurants. Healthcare executives need to refocus on their core business. The greater your product line, the less money, the fewer people, and the fewer resources are usually available for achieving market dominance in any one area.

The world of fast food offers another example of healthcare's need to stick to its core business. Bringing McDonald's fast-food fare into hospitals was a great marketing idea—for McDonald's! In reality, it was just another profit-driven healthcare oxymoron. Providing easy access to high-fat foods is counterproductive to a hospital's mission. It sends mixed messages about good eating habits and healthy lifestyles. Using retail strategies doesn't mean getting used by retailers.

CREATIVE COMMUNICATIONS

Of course you need to not only provide service that will distinguish you from your competitors, but you also need to *tell* your customers and potential customers about your services in a way that will make you distinct and original in their minds. This section addresses a range of communications techniques and strategies that will help achieve that goal.

Most healthcare brochures are me-too copycat designs. Your organization's marketing collateral (brochures, videos, etc.) needs to be unique, present a quality image, encourage action, and send a message that supports your branding. Design your marketing brochures using as many of the following guidelines as possible.

Reduce text and technical words.

Limit the text and do away with technical wording. Most people do not understand medical jargon. Consider, for example, a description of your efficient emergency room registration process. If you write "We have several nurses to assist with triage," what does this mean to the average person entering the emergency department? Perhaps nothing. Writing "to assist with check-in," however, would be better understood.

Use unique and interesting pictures of people.

Use pictures of people in action. Nobody wants to see your building unless it is critical to the decision process.

Maximize the advantages of color.

Research shows that color conveys quality and loyalty. People retain 40 to 50 percent more information from a color presentation (Peoples 1992).

Use words that sell.

Leaders are always trying to affect change, to persuade others, and to gain consensus. Your choice of words is important. A picture is worth a thousand words; however, the right word is worth a thousand pictures. Analyze advertising and direct mail pieces

THE 12 MOST PERSUASIVE WORDS

According to a Yale University study (Peoples 1992), the 12 most persuasive words in the English language are:

You	Results	Safety
Money	Easy	Have
Save	Healthy	Discovery
New	Guarantee	Proven

The four words in bold are the most powerful of the 12. You can become more persuasive by using these 12 words in all your communications. Consider the following sentence, which attempts the perhaps overly ambitious feat of using all 12 words.

When it comes to a *healthy* profit, *you* will *have* no difficulty *discovering* how *easy* and *safe* our *new* and *proven* technology is at generating *guaranteed money-saving results*.

Try incorporating these words into a sentence describing your organization, primary product, or service.

you receive: What words work and what words don't? Apply what works to your own advertising efforts.

To be more personal avoid using the words "we" and "I." Instead, exchange them for the word "you." Consider the following:

1. *We have multiple locations to serve you better.* (Typical)
2. *You will find one of our many locations most convenient.* (Better)

The second sentence is warmer, more personal, and emphasizes the patient benefit.

Design with the Golden Ratio.

The Golden Ratio, also known as the Golden Rectangular Ratio, is 1:0.618. Visuals constituting a height-to-width ratio of 1:0.618 are golden. Subconsciously, we like to see things with that ratio. Which of the following two rectangles do you prefer?

Rectangle A   **Rectangle B**

Chances are you picked rectangle "A" because its height to width ratio is at the golden ratio of 1:0.618. Use the golden ratio whenever possible when creating brochures, paragraphs, signage, photographs, forms, name tags, architectural design, classified ads, pictures, logos, employee badges, and advertising layouts.

Use a paper stock that will invoke a response.

Whenever possible use textured stock, embossing, and cutout areas to draw attention to your marketing collateral.

Present information, concepts, and items in groups of three-three-three.

Three is the magic number in our lives. People retain more information when it is presented in threes and are engaged by the rhythm of three. Give the reader three reasons for using your heart center, three reasons to be on time, three reasons to take their medication, and so on.

Audio and Video Brochures

Consider making a video or audio brochure to promote your medical staff, products, and services. Most people have an audio tape deck in their car and can listen to your message on the way to and from work, review what to expect on their first office visit, or go over the discharge and billing process with family members. Also consider an electronic brochure using interactive-voice-video-response (IVVR) technologies and putting your brochure on your web site. CD business cards and product brochures are available for promotions.

Telephone Cards

Provide specific patients or potential patients with a telephone calling card. Use these as access/intervention cards, perhaps to those who are at risk, depressed, or troubled.

Communications Collateral

Your organization is loaded with communication opportunities that might be passively going to waste. Consider how you can communicate your product and service excellence to your stake-holders using the following items:

- Business cards;
- Letterhead and envelopes;
- Checks and invoices;
- Business and clinical forms;
- Consultation reports;
- Couriers (person and uniform);
- Transportation and maintenance vehicles;
- Signage (internal and external);
- Fax cover page; and
- Web site.

Every document that leaves your facility is a branding opportunity and needs to carry a marketing message. The next time letterhead and envelopes are ordered, review their marketing message. Consider the following communications package for a full-service imaging center:

- Business cards are printed on both sides—the reverse side has a map and lists its imaging modalities;
- Letterhead and envelope carry the "Full-Service Imaging Center" tagline;
- Checks and invoices carry the "Full-Service Imaging Center" tagline;
- All business and clinical forms carry the "Full-Service Imaging Center" tagline;
- Consultation reports contain the "Full-Service Imaging Center" tagline and list all the modalities by name (e.g., MRI, CT, Ultrasound, Nuclear Medicine, General x-ray);
- Couriers' uniforms display appropriate information and the "Full-Service Imaging Center" tagline;

- Transportation and courier vehicles are imprinted with appropriate signage and the "Full-Service Imaging Center" tagline;
- All signage conforms to branding guidelines, is large enough to read at a distance, and is at eye level; and
- Fax cover page carries the "Full-Service Imaging Center" tagline and lists all the modalities.

Go through your organization and ensure that no branding and marketing opportunity is wasted. If something leaves the organization, the office, or the clinic, use the opportunity to exploit your branding and marketing message.

Fax Marketing

How are your fax machines being used in today's high-speed business environment? Still faxing consultation reports at an archaic rate? Upgrade your fax machines and speed up the process of doing business. Increase your company's name recognition with customers and referral sources by turning your fax machine into an education device. Start using your fax unit as a marketing tool. Consider faxing your customers the following documents:

- Healthcare updates;
- Managed care information;
- Product and service news;
- Operational changes;
- Productivity tips;
- Regulation and law updates;
- Special thank-you notes;
- Birthday greetings;
- Patient information;
- Invitations;
- Fax newsletters; and
- Personnel changes.

If done properly, your faxes can be a critical link to your customers. Note, however, that federal law prohibits unsolicited faxing of marketing, sales, or other information to prospects who have not specifically requested this information. Always secure a prospect's permission and your customer's approval before sending your first fax update.

Testimonials

Testimonials are a powerful way to bring a positive message to your customers. You should systematically collect testimonials from people who have had experiences with your organization, especially patients who have had a particularly favorable outcome. Place testimonials in a three-ring binder in waiting areas for patients to view or post them on a dedicated bulletin board in high-traffic areas.

Testimonials can also play an important role in your print communication. Consider featuring at least three testimonials in each issue of your newsletter and creating display advertising or direct-mail pieces based on testimonials. You could even create an audio or video promotion featuring several vivid testimonials.

Testimonials are not just for patients. You can share them— separately or through your newsletter—with physicians, managed care organizations, vendors, and community leaders.

You can even make use of negative testimonials. For example, you could post a negative testimonial along with how you resolved the problem. You can also use positive testimonials to combat negative perceptions. (Note: Make sure you get written authorization before using a person's testimonial or photograph.)

"Disconnect" Communications

An important place to communicate a positive message about your organization is during the "disconnect" process—when a patient is leaving your organization. This is your last chance to make a good impression, and it is an excellent opportunity to leave an impression that will stay with the patient. Effective disconnect communication might take the form of:

- a thank-you statement;
- a statement that staff has enjoyed serving the patient;
- a reassuring statement;
- a confirming statement;
- a statement about follow-up care;
- a warm, parting statement; and
- a statement about the patient's chosen provider.

Here is an example of a statement that could be made while a staff member is discharging a patient or taking her to awaiting transportation:

> "Ms. Brown, thank you for using Shaka General. We enjoyed having you here and serving your healthcare needs. You picked the right surgeon/hospital team to perform your surgery. We will call you in a few days to see how you are doing. Remember to call your doctor if you have any questions and concerns. Again, thank you for selecting Shaka General. If you or your family ever need medical care again, please keep us in mind, as we want to be your hospital of choice."

Direct Mail

You can stand out from your competitors with laser-like focus on three elements associated with direct mail. Those key elements, in order of importance, are:

1. The *list*—the focus and accuracy of prospect information that composes the mailing list;

2. The *offering*—response incentive to take immediate action; and
3. The *graphics*—the visual and verbal magnets that help draw the reader's interest.

Mailing lists are usually sold in thousand-name increments. One pays per thousand names, so a list of 5,000 names bought at a $65 per thousand-name rate costs $325. Many variables go into purchasing a list and how it is received—on a disk, as labels, etc. List companies "seed" their lists (i.e., include special "tracker" names and address). They employ those names and addresses to monitor how often the purchaser mails the list and to ensure that the list is only used for the purpose purchased. Some list companies and brokers require samples of the direct-mail piece(s) before providing the customer with a list, and then work with their clients to purchase the best mailing list from the abundant supply of list houses or companies. A list broker receives a brokerage fee, usually about 20 to 60 percent of the cost from the list company. As an example, if one purchases a list for $1,000, the list company will pay the broker $400. The customer pays the list broker indirectly through the list company.

See the list of tips (opposite) to help you ensure your direct-mail piece is effective, both in its message and its graphics, and that it does not share the destination of most direct-mail pieces: the trash.

MOVING AHEAD

This chapter has suggested strategies and techniques for ensuring that your organization is not a me-too provider—an organization perceived to offer the same services as most other organizations. The next chapter takes a look at a single strategy—branding. Its primary purpose is to distinguish your organization from its competitors.

TIPS FOR EFFECTIVE DIRECT-MAIL OFFERINGS

- Focus on the "power benefit" (the most important benefit) of the offer to get the reader's attention.
- Promise your power benefit in the headline or opening paragraph to maintain the reader's interest.
- Keep the reader excited by introducing one or two additional appealing benefits.
- Clearly link the desired actions in accepting your offer to the reader receiving each stated benefit.
- Maintain brevity; keep it simple and focused.
- Use one piece of paper for the direct-mail piece.
- Provide supportive information and materials *separately* from the main direct-mail piece.
- Use effective visuals—design, graphics, fonts, colors, photographs.
- Do not clutter the main direct-mail piece; use white space to open the piece up.
- Let the reader know exactly what products and services they are receiving by listing them.
- Back up all claims with proof using facts, reports, testimonials, and endorsements.
- Illustrate the benefits others have received.
- When using testimonials and endorsements use *their* words, not yours.
- Clearly define the reader's consequences for not executing specific desired action.
- Always include an emotional and enticing "act now or lose" message.
- Always impress a sense of urgency on the reader for taking specific action immediately.
- Close with a solid paragraph restating your offer and the reader's key benefits.
- Allow two weeks for dated response ("respond by . . .") offers, such as seminars, to reach a target group by mail.
- Keep improving your offer and the direct-mail piece presentation.

The Essence of Branding

BRANDING IS THE battle for the consumer's mind in becoming the provider of choice. Successful branding requires a solid, organized commitment to deliver unique standards of consistency as it relates to your products and services. Branding is the buzz that accelerates interest in your organization, both internally and externally. Conversely, indifference kills your efforts to create and maintain brand identification. The keys to effective branding are to:

- differentiate yourself from the me-too competition by breaking away from the pack;
- offer significant perceived value to win new customers and keep current ones;
- be aggressively proactive; and
- demand systemwide consistency.

Unless you break away from the me-too provider syndrome by branding, expect your business to turn into a commodity, where marketplace forces ask for more and pay less. And while your own brand identity is crystallizing, you must understand your competitor's brand image as well. This is crucial in differentiating yourself from the horde of me-too providers.

ESTABLISHING BRAND IDENTITY

Branding requires a systematic, consistent effort to embody your products and services within a clear identity and to communicate that identity to your stakeholders.

Deciding What to Brand

Deciding what to brand requires careful consideration of the services you offer, the people who provide the service, the competition's services, and the population you serve. For example, you might choose to brand:

- your entire health system;
- your outpatient service;
- a prominent department or medical program/procedure; or
- a luminary physician or medical group.

Consider brand concepts, products, and services that have a high demand but are difficult to emulate. For example, successful brands have been built around treating chronic conditions, providing women's health services, or providing geriatric services. As these examples show, effective brands are often, if not always, linked to specific target audiences such as women, men, seniors, or ethnic communities. The sidebar at the end of the chapter offers suggestions on marketing healthcare to one vitally important group: seniors.

Defining the Brand Message

Linked to a decision about what service to brand is a decision about what message you want to communicate about that service. You might decide to emphasize respect for patients, quality of care, convenience, high-tech capacity, or some other message that is especially resonant with your target audience and related to the service you are branding.

Communicating the Brand

A systemwide, multimedia strategic-communications campaign is necessary to introduce your brand message internally to your organization and externally to the community. In planning the campaign, consider the specific messages you need for both and then define "information dissemination" marketing channels for getting your message across. Make sure the overall message is clear, consistent, and continuous. Communication can take place through marketing collateral, business documentation, and advertising.

Energizing Employees

To make a brand successful, you need not only staff acceptance, but staff enthusiasm as well. Energize your employees to become both ambassadors of goodwill and salespeople. You can accomplish this by creating employee business units that take ownership of the branding communication efforts and by establishing rewards for staff involvement in the effort.

Fulfilling the Promise

Of course the true test of your brand is performance. You must ensure that every customer encounter entails lasting satisfaction, reinforces the brand identity, and is used as an opportunity to build a relationship with the customer. If you provide excellent service and educate your customers, they will turn into sources of new business. Remember, too, that when you think of customers, include end users, referral sources, and payers.

Collecting and Using Information

Information will be key to determining the performance of your brand, both as a healthcare service and as a customer service. You will need to create a systemwide computerized data collection, analysis, and reporting network that includes data about costs/financial performance of the brand, data about clinical outcomes related to the brand, and data about customers of the brand. Use this data continually to retool and market the brand.

Branding Proactively

Maintaining a thriving brand requires a strategy for proactive branding stewardship that effectively invigorates the branding process throughout the company, the community, and the customer base. Develop a branding action plan with visual icons and other distinctive attributes and methods to create a "brand buzz."

Protecting Your Brand

Protect your brand with patent and trademark rights for the brand itself, unique brand-building technologies, and significant differences between your brand and the competition's.

INTEGRATED MARKETING

Integrated marketing, also called cross-marketing, is the key to successful branding. It is a systemwide approach to marketing

products and services throughout any organization in our industry, including healthcare systems, physician networks, multi-
specialty practices, facility services, and multiple geographic
locations. To successfully integrate your marketing efforts,
you must:

- determine what you want to cross-market, including the
  brand's image, products and services, and branding strategy
  (including consistency in communication, product/service,
  and care).
- define the target customers, including physicians, patients,
  and family members of potential patients.
- determine systemwide customer contact points, including
  location (front desk, elevators, cafeteria, stairwells, waiting
  areas), medium (word-of-mouth, face-to-face), and staff.
- determine customer contact position, including volunteers,
  receptionists, and technologists.
- educate your customer-contact staff about the product or
  service, access process, and benefit.
- create appropriate marketing collateral, including message
  and medium (brochure, display advertising, and audiovisual
  advertising).
- survey target groups for effectiveness, including top-of-mind
  recall of the message and employees' opinion of effectiveness.

Successful integrated marketing requires organizationwide
participation, from top management down. You must walk the
talk or few others will follow.

MOVING AHEAD

With the background provided on marketing concepts, how to
distinguish yourself from your competitors, and branding, we
can move into more specific avenues of getting your message

out. The next chapter focuses on one of the hottest and most misunderstood techniques of marketing, not only in healthcare but in all business: Internet marketing.

MARKETING TO SENIORS

What to Avoid: Seven Myths About Seniors

Believing these myths about seniors will defeat your marketing efforts.

Myth One: People become "old" when they reach age 65.
In 1889, 65 was declared the age of the elderly by Prince Otto von Bismarck. Today, people 65 and older are more vital and active than ever.

Myth Two: Most older people are in poor health.
Aging may intertwine with illness, but quality of life need not suffer. According to the American Healthcare Association, only 5 percent of our nation's elderly reside in nursing homes.

Myth Three: Older minds are not as bright as young minds.
Only 10 percent of seniors show signs of memory loss and fewer than half of those show any serious mental impairment.

Myth Four: Older people are unproductive.
Older workers have fewer on-the-job injuries, fewer avoidable absences, and better attendance than their younger coworkers.

Myth Five: Older people are sexless.
Most older men and women enjoy sexual activity. Many find greater pleasure in sex as seniors than when they were young.

Myth Six: All older people are the same.
No age group varies more in physical abilities, personal styles, or financial capabilities than the senior population.

Myth Seven: Older people are out of touch with the world.
Thanks to their growing pursuit of continuing education, travel, and Internet access, seniors are rapidly becoming more sophisticated, especially where healthcare is concerned.

MARKETING TO SENIORS

> **What to Do: Insights on Marketing to Seniors**
>
> Golda Meir once said, "Old age is like an airplane flying through a storm. Once you're aboard, there's nothing you can do." Nevertheless, when marketing to seniors, there is a lot you can do. Consider the following key insights.
>
> - Seniors show a higher concern for quality over cost than consumers from all younger age groups.
> - Senior consumers want information that will allow them to take charge of their lives. Like most people, seniors want options in controlling their destiny.
> - Seniors have a greater concern for health and a growing fear over the limitations that a serious illness could cause.
> - Seniors most definitely want to retain their independence.
> - Seniors do not like to be thought of as old. Most seniors are not challenged by age. Society has just been misled to think that.
> - Seniors are more interested in purchasing experiences than things. Remember: Sell emotion first, logic second.
> - Seniors want convenience and easy access. It is integral to their independence.
> - Seniors typically base their buying decisions on security and safety—security in a quality product at a fair price, and safety while using the product.
> - Seniors want products and services that will make them feel and look better physically, mentally, and socially. Don't we all?
> - Seniors want to be comfortable, both physically and mentally.
>
> Figure 3.1 shows a range of marketing channels you can use to put these insights into action when marketing to seniors.

FIGURE 3.1   MARKETING CHANNELS FOR SENIORS

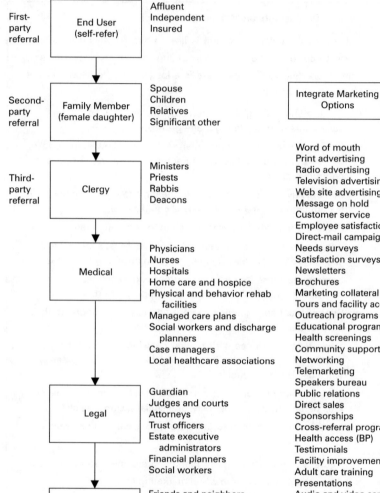

First-party referral	End User (self-refer)	Affluent Independent Insured
Second-party referral	Family Member (female daughter)	Spouse Children Relatives Significant other
Third-party referral	Clergy	Ministers Priests Rabbis Deacons
	Medical	Physicians Nurses Hospitals Home care and hospice Physical and behavior rehab facilities Managed care plans Social workers and discharge planners Case managers Local healthcare associations
	Legal	Guardian Judges and courts Attorneys Trust officers Estate executive administrators Financial planners Social workers
	Other	Friends and neighbors Current resident and support group Local clubs and civic groups Funeral home directors Adult day care administrators Employers and employees Competition Federal and state agencies Your employees and their family Vendors Visitors and service providers Health inspectors Retirement centers

Integrate Marketing Options

Word of mouth
Print advertising
Radio advertising
Television advertising
Web site advertising
Message on hold
Customer service
Employee satisfaction
Direct-mail campaign
Needs surveys
Satisfaction surveys
Newsletters
Brochures
Marketing collateral
Tours and facility access
Outreach programs
Educational programs
Health screenings
Community support
Networking
Telemarketing
Speakers bureau
Public relations
Direct sales
Sponsorships
Cross-referral program
Health access (BP)
Testimonials
Facility improvements
Adult care training
Presentations
Audio and video service
Facsimile (fax)
Information hotline
Compensation program
Special programs (ELC)
Volunteer program
Senior programs

4

Internet Marketing

MANY BELIEVE THE Internet is the one most significant influence changing the delivery of healthcare. The reason? We are digitizing, analyzing, and publicizing every aspect of the healthcare industry for the world to see. Every year, more people look to the Internet for up-to-date healthcare information. All of which suggests that your organization should have a presence on the Internet. You may wish to have a "bare-bones" web site with minimal information and interactive responses. However, if you have the time, money, and commitment, the Internet offers many options and opportunities for communicating with your customers and doing business. A wide array of potential healthcare uses for the Internet exists — uses you can incorporate into your own organization's web site.

A recent Deloitte Consulting-Cyber Dialogue study, "Cybercitizen Health 1999," offers valuable insight into what health-

POTENTIAL WAYS A HEALTHCARE ORGANIZATION CAN USE THE INTERNET

Staff education	Hospital selection
Preventative care	Physician selection
Healthcare information	Online support groups
Telemedicine	Emergency first aid
Previsit documentation and forms completion	Nursing home monitoring
	Facility tours
Newsletters	Health events calendar
Customer service	Volunteer scheduling
Patient surveys	Disease management
Directions and maps	Direct-mail prescription delivery
Direct complaint line	Personal care
Procedure information	Seniors program
Case management	Real-time observing (birthing, operations)
Plan enrollment	
Member services	Recruiting and interviewing
Free Internet access station for patients and family	Fundraising
	Community service
Marketing collateral (i.e., brochures)	Patient compliance monitoring
Patient education	
Reminder service	

related resources people are tapping into on the Internet, who is most likely to be seeking health information online, and what types of information they are seeking. Table 4.1 summarizes the results.

Those surfing the Internet for healthcare and medical information are doing so for their own or another's personal benefit. Clearly, the Internet is being used for second and third opinions as well. Online healthcare rankings, diagnosis-related

TABLE 4.1   USE OF THE INTERNET FOR HEALTH-RELATED
INFORMATION

Source of information sought on the Internet

Primary:		Secondary:	
1. Personal physician	62%	4. Insurers	45%
2. National experts	61%	5. Drug companies	42%
3. Hospitals	58%	6. Internet companies	42%
		7. Media companies	33%

Type of information sought over the Internet:

1. Specific conditions	73%	6. Fitness	36%
2. Diet and nutrition	49%	7. Children's health	30%
3. Pharmaceuticals	42%	8. Doctors	22%
4. Women's health issues	41%	9. Health insurance	14%
5. Alternative medicine	37%	10. Elderly care	13%

Source: Adapted from "Cybercitizen Health 1999." Deloitte Consulting-Cyber Dialogue.

chatrooms, medical data, and treatment information are turning once uninformed patients into knowledgeable, proactive ones who are just as informed as their doctors. The curtain of mystery that once veiled healthcare is parting. Patient access to the best practices, the best pharmaceuticals, and the best doctors will determine healthcare's future.

CREATING AN INTERNET PRESENCE

Establishing and managing a web site is a time-consuming and potentially expensive endeavor. To ensure that your site has a clear purpose, works toward that purpose, and is effectively and efficiently managed, you will need a systematic process. The following steps can be used to create a successful Internet presence.

1. Determine your primary goals and secondary objectives for having a web site presence, including:
   a. business objectives;
   b. healthcare objectives; and
   c. medical intervention objectives.
2. Create an Internet Production Team and appoint a team leader. Staff on the team should include representatives of the following functions and positions:
   a. marketing;
   b. finance;
   c. medical care;
   d. product and service managers;
   e. other (i.e. legal, risk management, business development staff); and
   f. web site specialist/consultant.
3. Determine your target audience(s) and customers.
4. Determine the type of web site presence you need—major or minor, hosted or outsourced—based on your goals, objectives, and target audience interactive response.
5. Determine the scope of products and services you want to promote on the Internet.
6. Determine the interactive-voice-vision-response (IVVR) medium to use for each product and service promoted on the Internet.
7. Identify legal and security issues and determine appropriate actions to address them.
8. As with any new product or undertaking, create a business plan for your web site, including:
   a. financials (resources, results, and revenue);
   b. web site staff, content, development, and implementation;
   c. how the web site will be marketed, both internally and externally; and

    d. how you will secure your web site domain name, also called the web site address or uniform resource locator (URL).

9. Determine Internet server, telephone line type, and service:
    a. host or outsource server; or
    b. existing standard telephone line or dedicated T-1 line.

10. Focus on creating an informative web site that is unique, memorable, easy to access and navigate, and has sustaining drawing power (measured in number of hits).

11. Create the web site in phases. Evolve, learn, and become more valuable as you go. You might implement the following services in this order:
    a. provide general information;
    b. offer specific products and services; and
    c. provide educational and self-help services.

12. Crash-test your web site before going online using internal and external users.

13. Educate your staff systemwide as to web site ownership, access, and content.

14. Educate the outside world and target customer markets and customers.
    a. Promote web site on all stationary, marketing collateral, documentation, advertising, etc.
    b. Actively list with search engines and periodically repeat listing.

15. Monitor, analyze, and revise to meet web site goals and objectives.

INTERNET COSTS

At this writing, you can own a web site domain (URL) for $35 per year. You can store or house your web site on an Internet service provider (ISP) for $50 to $100 a month, depending on the size and complexity of the site. Web page layout and graphic complexity directly dictates creative costs—the more interactive the web site, the more it costs to create. Expect to pay $500 to $2,500 to create a basic initial web site. Outsourcing the creation of a basic site with several simple pages typically costs between $1,000 and $2,000. Updates and maintenance will cost $100 to $2,000 per month. Figure in what it will cost to advertise your web site. Because revising your web site or page costs extra, consider purchasing an annual maintenance contract to take care of such things. Constructing, hosting, and maintaining a web site will total between $35,000 and $100,000 or more. A major (commercial) web site presence typically costs more than one million dollars annually.

MOVING AHEAD

The Internet is the most visible manifestation of what is often called the Information Age. This chapter has addressed how the Internet can help you convey information to customers. However, you also need to have information *about* your customers. The next chapter discusses how such information can be compiled, organized, and used to improve your competitive position.

5

Referral Database Mining

CUSTOMER KNOWLEDGE IS more important than product knowledge. Simply put, if you don't know and understand your customers, you will not be able to satisfy them. A database will help you to:

- identify customers and their interests and needs;
- manage your business better to meet those interests and needs;
- identify individual and industry referral trends;
- identify new business opportunities; and
- identify the best business (referral sources, procedures, and patients) to go after.

DATABASE DYNAMICS

A database can be compared to a filing cabinet where each drawer houses file folders and each folder stores information. The filing cabinet drawer acts as a database, albeit an inefficient one. The files are the individual records, and the types of information within the file folders are the record's fields. A field is the specific space within a record for putting information, such as a name, an address, a telephone number. Healthcare marketing needs access to three general types of databases.

1. A *customer* database that houses information about patients, payers, and physicians.
2. A *financial* database that houses information about products, costs, and revenues.
3. A *competitive* database that houses information about competitors' names, products/services, and pricing.

Unfortunately, most healthcare organizations have limited access to customer and competitive data. Instead, the business computer systems, related software, and data collection deal solely with financial information. Marketing people need customer information: the closer they get to your customers, the closer your customers get to the organization. The following nine steps provide direction toward becoming a data-driven organization, especially with regard to customers and competitors.

1. Define the purpose of the database.
2. Determine what data you need and where that data reside.
3. Collect data.
4. Create the database.
5. Enter the data into the database.
6. Mine the database by looking for key information, patterns, and trends.
7. Profile customer groups by searching for common traits.
8. Create reports oriented to the desired information.
9. Keep the database current.

The four sidebars at the end of the chapter offer examples of databases related to customers and competition, with suggested fields to help guide your database creation and maintenance.

CREATING PROFITABILITY PROFILES

Profitability profiling enables you to identify referral opportunities and focus on resources to maximize your return on sales and services. Without profiles, an organization is taking the same marketing approach for consumers, prospects, and customers. Marketing professionals need the following four profiles to help them with their strategic decisions, create better advertising, and focus their resources:

1. referral source;
2. patient;
3. managed care plan; and
4. employer.

As an example, consider the following scenario using the physician profile analysis format in Table 5.1. The marketing department releases a new service for physicians. They believe the ideal referrer is an orthopedist, age 55, a member of St. Peter's medical staff, and with an office within 15 miles of the hospital. The physician is the decision maker. After a few months, the marketing people query their database to profile their best referral source by profit and volume. The profile shows that the best referral source is a female general practitioner, age 45, practicing within seven miles of St. Peter's, a member of St. Barbara's medical staff, with a nurse as the decision maker. Armed with that profile, what should a salesperson do? Answer: Visit the nurses of female general practitioners, age 45, within seven miles of St. Peter's, and on staff at St. Barbara's.

TABLE 5.1   PHYSICIAN PROFILE ANALYSIS

No.	Characteristics	Ideal	Best	Typical
1	Age	55	**45**	50
2	Sex	M/F	**Female**	M/F
3	Specialty	Orthopedic	**GP & FP**	Mix
4	Location (within miles)	15m	**7m**	80% w/in 10m
5	Decision maker	Physician	**Nurse**	Office Mgr.
6	Medical staff (hospitals)	St. Peter's	**St. Barbara's**	St. Peter's

A profitability profile can also be created for the following areas by identifying common characteristics of your best:

• payer mix;
• procedure mix;
• patient mix;
• referral source mix;
• managed care plan mix;
• employer mix;
• vendors; and
• geographical areas.

Focus your marketing and selling efforts on those areas that show the greatest potential for return on sales and services (ROSS).

MAPPING DATA

To gain special insight about your service area, referrals, and the competition, consider mapping your data. By mapping data, either electronically or manually, you see things that are not evident by just analyzing the numbers. With mapping, you look for patterns. Some patterns are of strategic importance, explaining why desired business is not at expected levels. As a hypothetical example, a map showing dots for each patient might show that few Parkview Hospital patients cross Roosevelt Boulevard, a major multilane roadway. Mapping shows information that just scanning numbers may miss. Perhaps establishing a medical clinic on the other side of Roosevelt Boulevard would draw patients to the hospital.

Most data can be mapped to provide insightful information. The Dartmouth Atlas is a good example. It mapped Medicare information that suggests problems in the national delivery of quality healthcare. Consider mapping the following types of information:

- referral sources;
- patients;
- competitors;
- healthcare providers;
- procedures;
- bad debts;
- diseases; and
- dissatisfied patients.

Mapping is readily accomplished by using one of the many inexpensive mapping software programs that work with databases.

GRAPHING DATA TO GAIN INSIGHT

Consider graphing referral and other data to better see anomalies. Graphs convey information quicker than endless rows of numbers. As an example, in the following physician monthly referral report (Table 5.2), physicians are sorted by name. The referral information provided includes physicians' projected year-end (PYE) referrals. Use the equation @sum/@count × 12 to calculate a projected year-end on any spreadsheet program. The PYE is a valuable number to know for planning purposes.

TABLE 5.2 PHYSICIAN MONTHLY REFERRAL REPORT (ALPHABETICAL SORT)

Name	TYP	SP	Jan	Feb	Mar	Apr	May	Jun	Jul	Aug	Sep	Oct	Nov	Dec	YTD	PYE	LYT	VAR
Austin	MD	GP	3	4	3	5	2	6	1	1	3	5			33	40	32	24
Bears	MD	GP	12	11	13	12	15	16	12	5	12	14			122	146	145	1
Cabin	MD	FP	6	7	7	7	8	6	7	2	8	9			67	80	79	2
Dock	**DO**	**INT**	**22**	**21**	**18**	**19**	**15**	**12**	**9**	**3**	**5**	**5**			**129**	**155**	**125**	**24**
Eagles	DC	CHI	2	2	2	2	2	2	4	1	5	7			29	35	36	(3)
Frogger	MD	Psych	8	11	9	4	7	12	3	1	4	7			66	79	68	16
Gilmore	MD	Orto	1	1	1	1	1	1	2	1	4	6			19	23	22	44
Hooks	MD	BP	11	13	12	11	11	12	13	8	13	15			119	143	125	14
Inlets	MD	GYN	4	3	8	5	2	5	9	2	4	9			51	61	45	36
Joy	MD	GP	27	19	26	26	25	32	29	30	28	32			284	341	195	75
Totals	10		96	102	99	92	88	104	89	54	86	109	0	0	919	1103	872	19

FIGURE 5.1 PHYSICIAN REFERRALS BY MONTH

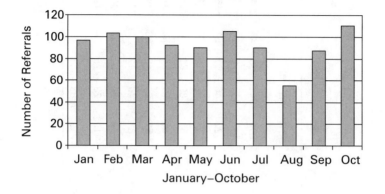

Notice that, year-to-date (YTD), Dr. Dock's variance (VAR) from last year's total (LYT) shows a gain of 24 referrals. However, if one looks at the monthly referral pattern, it clearly suggests an area of concern. Always investigate variances and deviations.

Compare the aggregate monthly referrals, as shown in both the physician monthly referral record in Table 5.2 and the graph in Figure 5.1, and decide which best shows a referral pattern. Notice the major referral dip in August. Such a dip may be the result of many referral sources going on vacation simultaneously. By similarly comparing three or more years' monthly referrals by graphing each year on the same chart, one will see their cyclic referral pattern, their work load, and their operating demands. When a major dip is present, turn the slack time into an opportunity. This may be the best time for your employees to take their vacations, receive training, or do strategic planning. Do not compromise access, service, and quality during premier business cycles (high patient loads) by permitting staff to take vacations, engage in off-site training and meetings, conduct health screenings, etc., at these prime times.

In Table 5.3, the same physicians are now sorted by volume. The key things to note in this report are the aggregate referrals—

TABLE 5.3   PHYSICIAN MONTHLY REFERRAL REPORT (VOLUME SORT)

Name	TYP	SP	Jan	Feb	Mar	Apr	May	Jun	Jul	Aug	Sep	Oct	Nov	Dec	YTD	PYE	LYT	VAR		
Joy	MD	GP	27	29	26	26	25	32	29	30	28	32			284	341	233	46	284	29
Dock	DO	INT	22	21	18	19	15	12	9	3	5	5			129	155	125	24	413	42
Bears	MD	GP	12	11	13	12	15	16	12	5	12	14			122	146	97	51	535	54
Hooks	MD	BP	11	13	12	11	11	12	13	8	13	15			119	143	110	30	654	66
Cabin	MD	FP	6	7	7	7	8	6	7	2	8	9			67	80	80	1	721	73
Frogger	MD	Psych	8	11	9	4	7	12	3	1	4	7			66	79	84	(6)	787	80
Inlets	MD	GYN	4	3	8	5	2	5	9	2	4	9			51	61	45	36	838	85
Austin	MD	GP	3	4	3	5	2	6	1	1	3	5			33	40	12	230	871	88
Eagles	DC	CHI	2	2	2	2	2	2	4	1	5	7			29	35	32	9	900	91
Gilmore	MD	Orto	1	1	1	1	1	1	2	1	4	6			19	23	25	(9)	919	93
Totals	10		96	102	99	92	88	104	89	54	86	109	0	0	919	1103	843	41		

FIGURE 5.2   PHYSICIAN MONTHLY REFERRALS (RANKED BY VOLUME)

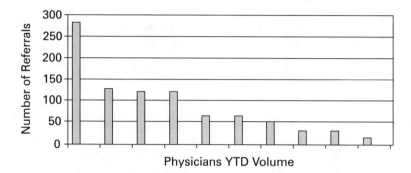

that is, the top referring physician added to the next highest, and so on. The top three referral sources account for 54 percent of all referrals. Under this scenario, this business is on shaky ground. If anything happens to any one of the top three referral sources, the business probably cannot recuperate from the losses. Figure 5.2 shows the physicians' YTD volume as a graph. See how quickly graphing shows the relationships.

MOVING AHEAD

So far, this book has focused primarily on marketing to individuals, including individual consumers and physicians. Of course these are not the only sources of patients and revenue for your organization. Especially in the current climate, payers are a crucial customer and target of your marketing efforts. The next chapter looks at how you market to managed care plans and how to create favorable relationships with those plans.

PHYSICIAN DATABASE

The following information could constitute a physician database. Most of this information can be gleaned from medical directories, professional organizations, telephone directories, and other readily available resources.

Name
Doctor type (MD, DO, DC)
Specialty
   Subspecialty
Sex
Age
Date of birth
Personality type
Religious preferences
Ethnic affiliation
   Language(s)
Practice type (Solo/Group)
   Partners' names
Primary address
   Secondary address
Home address
Telephone number(s)
   Fax number(s)
Hospital affiliations
MCO provider panel(s)
Employer affiliation(s)
Office hours
   Best time to call
   Day off
   In surgery
Office staff—bios
Personality type
   Office manager
   Nurse(s)
   Physician assistant
   Receptionist
   Billing clerk
   Other
Spouse's name (occupation)
   Children
   Family pet(s)
Vacation(s)

Holidays observed
Business(s) ownership(s)
Professional interests
Personal interests / hobbies
Associations membership
   Current / past offices held
License number
Medical school
   Year graduated
   Class ranking
   Internship(s)
Key relationships / influence
   Political
   Medical
   Physician
   Community
   Company
Date of first referral
Referral motivation
Referral volume per month
Referral payer mix
Referral procedure mix
Referral ranking
Gross revenue
Profitability ranking
Special requests
Automobile type
Assigned territory / cluster
   Travel time / distance
   Parking / costs
Lunch preferences
General likes and dislikes
Sales representative
Sales call frequency
Date of last sales call
Follow-up action
Comments

PATIENT DATABASE

The following patient data is invaluable to marketing people, especially when trying to generate new patients.

Name	Personal physician status
Age	Name(s)
Sex	Referral source
Ethnic group	Primary
Religious affiliation	Secondary
Address	Procedure(s)
City	Transportation
State	Head of household
Zip Code	Hospital preference
Telephone number	Visit frequency
Marital status	Date of first visit
Income level	Date of last visit
Education level	Personal interests
Occupation	Community interests
Employer	Influence level
Work telephone number	Community
Medical benefits	Business
Insurance-payer mix	Political
Insurance plan coverage	Media mix
Deductible	Television
Copayment	Radio
Family structure	Paper
Healthcare decision maker	Magazine
Spouse	Relationship to other patients
Occupation	Membership(s)
Employer	Organizations
Education level	Comments
Family members	
Sex	
Age	

MANAGED CARE PLAN DATABASE

The following data has many uses such as negotiating contracts. Consider petitioning the local library to provide managed care directories, hospital directories, and healthcare newsletters to gain free access to them. Many other resources are available on the Internet.

Plan name	Date contract received
Parent company / owners	Date contract signed/returned
Local address	Date contract activated
City	Date contract renews/expires
State	Market share (%)
Zip Code	Market strategy
Telephone numbers	Three-year enrollment trend
Fax numbers	Projected growth rate
Corporate address	Geographical coverage
Primary contact(s)	Access points
Administrative executive(s)	MCO's financial rating
Case manager (UR-PR)	Claim account-receivable days
Provider contracting	Denial ratio per 1000 claims
Medical director (phy. profile)	Authorization requirements
MCO type (HMO, PPO, IPA)	POS options
MCO specialty (med, dental, WC)	Deductible(s)
Reimbursement type (cap, FFS)	Contracted services
Corporate type (profit–nonprofit)	Negotiated discount(s)
Number of insured lives (date)	Key providers
Number of providers	Gatekeeper system
Directory updated	Strengths / weaknesses
Date MCO started	Accreditation status
Contract under evaluation	HMO rating (if HMO)
Profitability by	Claim and data transmission
Plan	Comments
Procedure	
Physician	

COMPETITOR DATABASE

Create a competitor database and mine its content for strategic information. The following competitor database is basic, but it offers a sound starting point. If your competition is a publicly traded company, owning one share of stock will give you access to corporate information reserved for shareholders, including various reports, access to their Internet site, and other important benefits.

Name	Competitive threat
Location	Primary
Office type	Secondary
National	Service areas
Regional	Territories
Local	Products / services
Address	Price
Parent company name	Delivery
Private	Marketing strategy
For-profit	Sales force
Nonprofit	Size
Address	Compensation
Telephone number/Fax number	Training
E-mail address	Marketing collateral
Web site address	Brochures
Operations	Advertising / promotional
V-M-V	Placement
Service	Budget
Financial	Response strategy
Manufacturing	Strengths
Engineering (clinical)	Weaknesses
Product research	Opportunities
Product development	Comments

6

Gaining Managed Care Business

THE MORE YOU manage your own managed care business, the less managed care plans will manage you. What follows are proven tips for marketing to managed care plans and maximizing your managed care business.

MANAGED CARE'S PRIORITIES

Insurance companies are under constant pressure to improve financial performance for their shareholders. In general, managed care organizations have pursued these goals by attempting to control access to care, measuring and managing utilization, measuring and managing patient care processes and outcomes, pricing competitively, and contracting selectively for Medicare and Medicaid business.

61

In these efforts, managed care organizations work with providers who use the most cost-effective means to provide the best outcomes in the shortest period of time. To be successful in a managed care market, providers must pursue these goals as well because they are what the customer—in this case, the managed care organization—wants.

To be profitable, the most important thing a managed care plan requires from its provider panel (business partners) is a significant reduction in the plan's operating costs without compromising quality. This can be achieved by:

- reducing total delivery costs—do what you do less expensively without compromising quality.
- lowering costs per discharge—ensure that your treatment process conforms to accepted standards, best practices, scientifically based medicines, and benchmark outcomes.
- lessening member/patient encounter costs—do it right the first time, so the member/patient does not have to return unnecessarily.
- cutting their internal *customer* service costs—make it easy for managed care plans to conduct business with you by not letting your internal shortcomings become their costly problems. Dealing with a healthcare provider needs to be seamless.

When managed care organizations and providers part company, it is most often over issues related to cost and quality. In addition, a plan might drop a provider because of a change in the network or the inability to provide desired geographic coverage.

The sections that follow suggest methods for showing a managed care organization that your organization can help support the payer's goals.

CREATING A MANAGED CARE BROCHURE

A healthcare provider's brochure will best serve decision makers by providing information typically required by most managed care organizations and employers. When creating your managed care brochure, consider including the following information:

- Organizational structure—ownership and operating history
- Accreditation status—accrediting organization, level or type of accreditation, and years of accreditation
- Management team—names, education, and experience
- Personnel—background, bonding, in-service training, and key staff members
- Financial history—financial solvency
- Services—range, continuum, products, and subcontracting
- Geographical coverage—offices, service facilities, sites, and map
- Emergency service capabilities—response staff, services, policies, and time
- Quality control—OSHA, systems, standards, and programs
- Training programs—managed care staff, community, and patients
- Provider relationships—current managed care contracts, employers, and physician-hospital organizations
- Guarantees—return-goods policy and procedure and service guarantees
- Utilization review and risk management—policies, systems, and programs
- Billing and collections—policies, procedures, software programs, and systems
- Performance measurement and improvement—data collection and use related to utilization, patient satisfaction, cost, outcomes, and systems

- Communication technology—system interfacing, site linking, and scheduling
- Customer service—patient satisfaction program, including monitoring and addressing issues

The person responsible for an organization's managed care business and compliance needs the above information in greater detail than one expects to find in a brochure. This information also needs to be placed in a three-ring binder as a reference, especially for negotiations. Having a dedicated managed care person is critical to maximizing your managed care business and profits.

MANAGED CARE CONTRACTING TIPS

The following contracting tips will greatly enhance your ability to negotiate a beneficial managed care contract.

Create your own "negotiate to" boilerplate managed care contract. Using your top-three managed care plan contracts that generate the most revenue, most volume, and the least hassle, create a boilerplate reference contract comprising the best terms and conditions from the three contracts. Negotiate every managed care contract to your boilerplate reference. The more boilerplate terms and conditions you negotiate into a managed care contract, the better your chances of having a desirable outcome.

Request the top three reasons why the plan rejects submitted claims.
Make sure everyone knows the most common reasons claims are rejected, and put safeguards in place to lessen the chances of committing those errors in the claim process. You want to reduce managed care plan claim-floating tendencies, while speeding up your reimbursement payments.

Request a sample "clean" claim for the top revenue-producing procedures.
Have each managed care plan provide a sample "clean" claim—that is, one completed with all the right codes, modifiers, and other information needed to process a claim successfully. Include the same as a contract addendum.

Determine the cost to sign a managed care contract.
Review each separate terms-and-conditions paragraph of the contract for its administrative and financial effect on the organization. Determine if additional staff, new computer work stations, software programs, tables, chairs, filing cabinets, etc., are required. Convert your needs to dollars.

Include a retroactive negotiating clause for contract revisions.
Include a clause that requires all contract revisions to be retroactive from the beginning of the contract. This is to everyone's benefit, especially if a managed care plan has underpaid a capitated per-member per-month premium.

Avoid a "favored nation" clause on their behalf.
Avoid this type of clause, which basically states that if a managed care plan negotiates a specific price with a provider and that provider turns around and offers another managed care plan or entity a lower price, the first managed care plan is entitled to the lower price, retroactively.

Display deductible and copayment office signage.
Appropriately display office signage declaring that federal law requires the collection of all Medicare beneficiaries' deductibles and copayments by the healthcare provider and that managed care contracts require the same from participating providers.

Set a deadline for the plan to request an adjustment.
Establish a reasonable time period—180 days—for a managed care plan to request and make an adjustment.

Require all adjustments of payment or overpayment refunds to be made in writing.
Establish that all adjustments of payments and overpayment refunds be made in writing and that each is substantiated in writing along with the original request. Bar plans from taking unilateral offsets. State that your written permission is required to take an offset.

Request an overall payment-dispute resolution process.
Suggest an overpayment-dispute resolution process. Avoid third-party arbitration, especially if it takes away your right to pursue resolution in the courts.

WORKING A NEW MANAGED CARE CONTRACT

You have signed the managed care contract and start to wonder where the referrals are. Managed care plans seldom spend any effort advertising and promoting one specific provider over another. Therefore, you must take an aggressive initiative to promote your organization as the provider of choice to potential referral sources within managed care plans. The flow chart in Figure 6.1 highlights a proven process for maximizing managed care contract referrals. To properly work a new or existing managed care contract, follow these guidelines.

1. Secure the managed care plan's latest provider directory and review its directory panels against your current referral source base (those physicians who already refer to your organization).
2. Create two referral source lists:
   a. an "A" list of referral sources that currently refer to your organization and are included on the managed care plan's panel; and

   b. a "B" list of those physicians on the managed care plan that have never referred to your organization (potential referral sources).

3. Contact those on the "A" list first because they already have a relationship with your organization. The rule of thumb is to contact six times in thirty days, by telephone, letter, postcard, fax, e-mail, or in person.

4. Review the "B" list with all those on the "A" list.

5. Solicit a referral from the "A" list to see someone on the "B" list.

6. Contact those on the "B" list, using the "six times" rule.

7. Ask the managed care plan for the names of their top utilizers for the services you offer. Contact those high utilizers first; therefore, if you provide MRI services, ask for the names of those physicians that order the most MRIs.

FIGURE 6.1   "WORKING" A MANAGED CARE CONTRACT

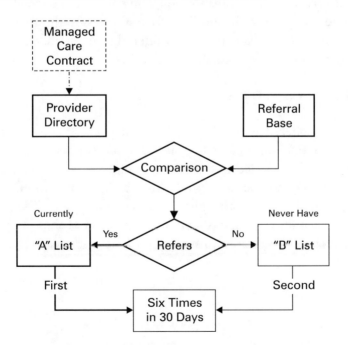

Another helpful tool for working with a managed care plan is a matrix of key information. Such a matrix is critical to increasing cash flow, claim acceptance, and referral source relationships. Start by making a table that includes the following information:

- managed care plan name;
- key contact people;
- telephone number(s);
- fax number(s);
- subplans;
- services covered (and *not* covered);
- member/patient deductible;
- member/patient copayment;
- required authorizations;
- special directives; and
- comments.

Everyone in your organization who comes into contact with a referral source and patient needs easy access to this managed care matrix. Give a copy to your referral sources; after all, they can use the same information.

MOVING AHEAD

The tips offered in this chapter should help you secure managed care contracts and make the most of those contracts once you secure them. Added to the other chapters so far in this book, you should now have a strong sense of how to communicate your organization's strengths to the key customers. The next section of the book focuses on another aspect of showing your organization's strengths in such a way that customers make the best use of your services: sales.

SECTION TWO

Sales

7

Sales and Selling Systems

MANY HEALTHCARE PROVIDERS, hospital administrators, and managers believe selling is simply having an employee socialize and tell others about their products and services. As a result of this common misconception, valuable consumers, customers, and referral sources are lost to the competition. Telling is not selling. As we explore the sales and selling processes involved in establishing a healthcare-based sales organization, the differences will become very apparent. But to help, compare the following differences between marketing and sales.

A SALESPERSON BY ANY OTHER NAME

Everyone sells. Some just do not know it. Everyday you sell yourself, your reputation, your trust, your ideas, and your relationships to others. Many professionals (e.g., physicians) passively market

Marketing	versus	Sales
Thinking		Action
Message		Delivery
Macro		Micro
Strategic		Tactical
Planning		Execution
Goal		Results
Office		Field
Projection		Rejection
Cost		Revenue
Analysis		Insight
Idealistic		Pragmatic
Subjective		Objective
Perception		Reality
"Forest"		"Trees"

and sell their products and services based primarily on their past reputation. However, within a given market, the more competition for a finite consumer or end-user group (e.g., patients), the more important are sales and selling skills. Healthcare professionals have a historic aversion toward sales and selling. In fact, a salesperson by any other name is still a salesperson. Selling is the business of helping people help themselves succeed. Following are a few of the more accustomed names used in healthcare sales:

- Detail person (pharmaceutical)
- Sales representative
- Business development specialist
- Physician relations specialist
- Community relations coordinator
- Product and services consultant
- Referral specialist

- Referral acquisition coordinator
- Product line salesperson
- Diagnostic imaging specialist
- Customer relations coordinator and
- Marketing representative

THE FIVE "A"s OF SELLING

As a healthcare executive, you need to understand sales and selling dynamics. Increasing competition from me-too providers dictates that organizations must exploit all customer (revenue) acquisition, retention, and cultivation opportunities. If you want your sales team to excel, have them focus on the following five "A"s of successful selling.

1. Customer *Application*. Find and create applications for your products and services that help customers do what they do better.
2. Cost-to-Change *Analysis*. Convey to the customer the benefit-to-change for using your products and services. Also stress the benefit-*not*-to-change once the customer starts using your products and services.
3. Competitive *Advantage*. Show the competitive advantage the customer gains in increased profitability and market dominance by using your products and services.
4. Corporate *Assurance*. Demonstrate your company's commitment to the highest level of customer service. Promise that your company will be around to meet the customer's future needs.
5. Customer *Acceptance*. Deliver your products and services in a quality and price package that consistently meets or exceeds the customer's expectations.

SALESPERSON'S RESPONSIBILITIES

The following are the basic responsibilities that every salesperson and sales team must execute with efficiency and consistency.

- Prospecting: Searching for new consumers, business opportunities (referrals), and qualified prospects.
- Questioning and listening: Determining a potential customer's interests, desires, and needs.
- Offering enhancement options: Providing prospects with product and service options that support the benefit-to-change.
- Post-referral follow-up: Ensuring that your organization appropriately delivers its products and services to fulfill the customer's expectations on a continuous basis.
- Customer base maintenance: Reducing lost business from referral-base erosion.
- Marketplace feedback: Proactively observing, listening, and learning marketplace dynamics, needs, and influential trends.

You must never lose sight of the minimal responsibilities of your sales organization and its salespeople.

SELLING CYCLE

Every salesperson encounters the same selling process consisting of three distinct selling stages. First, salespeople represent themselves. Within five to seven seconds, a potential customer will decide whether or not they like your sales representative. Second, salespeople represent their organization or company. Positive representation of image, reputation, and service leads to great selling success. Third, salespeople represent an organization's enhancement or solution options third. This is the "close"—

how the organization can help others help themselves become successful at what they do.

THE CORE SELLING PROCESS

The core process that all selling concepts are based on is actually very simple. It involves getting the prospect's *attention* by identifying a need or problem, generating an *interest* in your product, creating a *desire* for the product (i.e., the enhancement or solution), developing *conviction* in the decision maker, and *closing* by asking the prospect for his or her business.

Attention

Establish a rapport with the prospect. The objective is to quickly gain the attention of the referral source and use this "state of attention" to progress to the next phase in the selling process. Remember, the "state of attention" can rapidly disappear, so do not waste time once you have captured it. You want to develop rapport with the decision maker; you want them to like you. People do business with people they like!

Interest

Build on the prospect's interests, desires, and problems. The decision maker's interests can be discovered or created. Ask probing, open-ended questions, and then listen carefully. Convert the interest into a need. Present that need back to the prospect as an enhancement or a problem that you can solve.

Desire

Create a strong want in the mind of the decision maker by painting "word-pictures" that clearly establish the benefits to be gained. Create desire for your organization's products based on the prospect's problem (converted interest).

Conviction

Resolve all obstacles and objections. Although the salesperson has created desire, the decision maker needs to be convinced that using your service is in his or her best interest. In this step, all objections and concerns are removed, allowing both the decision maker and salesperson to move forward to the last step in the selling process: the close.

Close

Ask for a verbal commitment to do business. Once the decision maker is solidly convinced that using your company's products is the right solution, ask for referrals. The close step is simply asking for referrals. In the event the decision maker was moved along without proper involvement to the selling process, the salesperson may have to go back to a previous step and proceed selling forward to the close again. As the salesperson moves through the selling process with the decision maker, the need to frequently "trial close" is necessary. Trial closing is the process of keeping the decision maker involved, by indirectly asking for his or her opinion and referrals. A trial closing brings the referral source closer to the actual closing—the act of referring. Following are some examples of trial closing statements designed to seek the prospect's opinion.

- "Would you use a laboratory that has your patient's test results on your desk within the same day?"
- "Do you prefer to operate on Wednesday or Thursday morning next week?"
- "Do you feel comfortable referring one of your patients to our facility today?"

- "Are you saying that the provider who meets your pricing needs will be given an exclusive service contract?"

In each case, the trial close keeps the decision maker involved with the selling process by asking the prospect's opinion and reinforcing his or her own convictions to use your services. Depending on the response of the decision maker, the salesperson knows where they stand in the selling process. An attempt at a trial close may lead to the actual close or a referral or establish the next step in the selling process.

Remember, the referral process, just like buying, is guided by emotion. The decision maker must pass through all five basic selling steps, often without realizing it, before he or she is ready to accept your products and services.

A MORE DETAILED PROCESS

Within the core sales process just outlined is a more detailed process by which sales people identify prospects, convince them of your services' value, and close the deal. That process can be broken down into the following steps (see Figure 7.1).

1. *Research.* Research involves collecting consumer, competition, and customer information and learning about your prospects and their industries.
2. *Prospecting.* Prospecting means finding potential customers from prospective consumer bases, as well as contacting—usually by telephone—and meeting with prospects.
3. *Sales call.* This step could be a new (cold) call or a call on an established prospect. This call requires the most intensive use of interpersonal skills. At this stage, the salesperson must question, listen, and learn, generating information about a customer's needs and motivation. The salesperson must determine the customer's interest in the organization's

services and must present the benefits to the customer based on the customer's needs. The salesperson must also address objections that might arise. Throughout this process, the salesperson must begin to build a relationship with, and build a commitment from, the customer. And, when necessary, the salesperson must also know how to accept rejection within a positive context.

FIGURE 7.1   THE SALES PROCESS

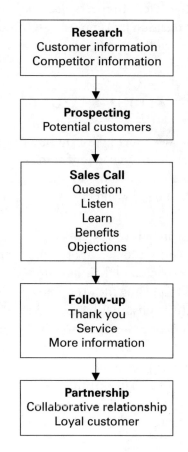

4. *Follow-up.* Follow-up begins with a thank you for the person's time and business. Follow-up also involves ensuring that the commitments you have made are kept, getting feedback about what your organization can do better, and letting customers know about changes and enhancements in your offerings. Effective follow-up will increase a customer's use of your services.

5. *Partnership.* Partnership is the goal of the salesperson-customer relationship. Achieving a partnership begins with building a cordial and then mutually respectful relationship, followed by a true collaborative relationship and a loyal customer.

MOVING AHEAD

Selling is an organizationwide effort. To be successful, it requires that everyone in the healthcare organization, system, and network focus, with dedication and enthusiasm, on creating and providing high-quality, unique, creatively delivered, reliable service. In turn, this service will create partnerships with loyal customers. These goals will not be achieved, however, without senior executive support—the super glue of sales.

The next chapter will show how to develop and retain effective salespeople who can carry out the basics outlined in this chapter.

8

Creating and Managing
Great Salespeople

FOR SALES EFFORTS to be successful, healthcare executives need to provide support to their salespeople. This chapter shows you how to support your sales staff through planning, communication, improving sales techniques, and compensation.

Above all, you can support your salespeople by treating them like professionals, understanding the fundamental process of sales, providing high-quality training, participating in sales activities when possible, keeping them up-to-date on the organization and the healthcare field, getting their input about customers and services, streamlining their paperwork and other work processes, and rewarding desired performance.

PLANNING

A concrete plan is necessary to turn vague marketing objectives into specific terms and actions. Such a plan is important for executives and for individual salespeople who can create and maintain their own plans. Figure 8.1 is a sample sales action plan that you can use as a model for your own plans.

Of course, you also need to be kept apprised of how the sales staff is progressing toward their goals. The three sales performance results reports in Figures 8.2 through 8.4 will keep you informed and provide valuable insight into your sales team's progress. Consider using the entity matrix in Figure 8.2 to report macro sales information by organization, department, sales team, territory, and individual salespeople. The sales force matrix in Figure 8.3 is great for reporting sales information by a specific referral source set, individual referral source, and customers overall. Use the best business opportunities matrix in Figure 8.4 for reporting a salesperson's or sales team's prospecting progress. By restructuring the tables, it is possible to report information by product line, service, salesperson, territory, etc.

SALES AUTOMATION

Another aspect of planning is to establish processes that will help your salespeople thrive. Perhaps the greatest opportunity for streamlining the day-to-day activities of sales is through automation. Sales force automation is more than equipping your salespeople with computers. Handing out notebook computers and contact/appointment software to your salespeople is not going to miraculously increase sales volume or productivity. Try implementing the following tips to automate sales processes successfully.

- *Assess manual processes.* Before automating, ensure that your current manual processes are adequate, effective, and working well. You do not want to automate a flawed system. If, however, you are using a proven "off-the-shelf" system,

FIGURE 8.1   SALES ACTION PLAN STATUS SHEET

Marketing Objective	Sales Macro (Strategies)	Sales Micro (Tactics)	Status (Results)
Increase managed care business by 20 percent by December	Increase managed care business by 10 percent in the 2nd Qtr, 5 percent in the 3rd Qtr, and 5 percent in the 4th Qtr		12 percent increase in 2nd Qtr 15 percent increase in 3rd Qtr
	Contact the ten largest managed care plans in service area	Contact and meet with the following managed care plan decision makers by March: HealthMed, Inc MetLife Aetna United Physicians USA Healthcare FirstChoice BlueCare Health Network Maxicare Health Trust	 Completed 1/30 Completed 2/05 Completed 2/21 Completed 2/06 Completed 2/13 Completed 2/13 Completed 2/03 Completed 2/26 Completed 3/11 Completed 3/03
	Schedule meetings with decision makers for each plan	Customize a managed care presentation by January 15 for each plan	Completed 1/10
	Make formal presentations to each decision maker	Determine interests and needs for each plan	Completed 3/15
		Develop individual sales strategy for each plan	Completed 4/01

FIGURE 8.2   SALES PERFORMANCE RESULTS BY ENTITY (SALESPERSON, TERRITORY, OR COMPANY)

	Month(s)	Year to Date	Projected Year-End	Last Year YTD	Variance
Forecasted Actual	Units/ Dollars	Units/ Dollars	Units/ Dollars	Units/ Dollars	Units/ Dollars
Variance					
Product AA≅					
Product AB≅					
Product A etc.≅					

FIGURE 8.3   SALES PERFORMANCE RESULTS BY REFERRAL SOURCE (PRODUCT/SERVICE, TERRITORY, OR SALESPERSON)

	Month(s)	Year to Date	Projected Year-End	Last Year YTD	Variance
Forecasted Actual	Units/ Dollars	Units/ Dollars	Units/ Dollars	Units/ Dollars	Units/ Dollars
Variance					
Product AA≅					
Product AB≅					
Product A etc.≅					

FIGURE 8.4   SALES PERFORMANCE RESULTS BY BEST BUSINESS OPPORTUNITIES (PRODUCT LINE, TERRITORY, OR SALESPERSON)

Prospect	Product/Service	Target Sale	Current Status	Close Strategy
a. Name	Name	Units/Dollars		
b. Name				

you may not need as thorough an assessment of your current processes.

- *Establish agreement.* Gain agreement between salespeople and management that information exchange between both parties is a "win-win-win" scenario: the salesperson wins, the company wins, the customer wins.
- *Establish the key elements of sales automation.* Explore all the key elements composing sales automation. Those elements include:

  — customer feedback;
  — customer profiling database;
  — customer and appointment log;
  — product problems;
  — current pricing information;
  — generating quotations;
  — qualifying guidelines;
  — activity and expense reporting;
  — product information; and
  — shipping information and status.

- *Establish an automation budget.* Typically, you can expect to pay about $1,500 for a desktop computer and $2,500 for a laptop. Estimate software to range between $150 and $5,000 per salesperson and training to be two to three times the cost of the hardware and software combined. And don't forget upgrades, maintenance, and the cost of insuring field computers.
- *Establish an effective training program.* Automation efforts often fail because the sales force has a problem operating the equipment and/or software. Your training program must be sufficient to instill confidence in using the computer and software. Post-training field support is critical to maintain the sales force's confidence.

- *Inputting and retrieving.* Inputting and retrieving data must be easy to do. Simplify the process and determine the best way to enter data on the computer screen. Consider access control, read/write/download authority, and termination of access issues.
- *Firmly establish financial incentive.* Your salespeople must perceive the personal value of automation in helping them achieve their financial objectives. Implanting that message will create a strong incentive to learn and use the new system.
- *Identify a reputable automation specialist.* Enlist a professional to help your team of marketing, sales, management, service, and support department representatives. A specialist can define your needs, introduce you to automation, suggest equipment, assist with training, and maintain the sales automation.

Efficiently putting important data and key systemwide information at the disposal of your salespeople is the optimal ending in sales automation. This goes beyond contact management automation.

EDUCATION AND RESOURCES

As a leader, you should be able to hire the best people for your sales force and to help the force continuously improve. The following are the core characteristics that you want to see in your new hires and that you want to instill through education in your current sales staff:

- Recognizes and takes advantage of opportunity
- Resourceful with limited resources
- Creative, not an imitator
- An independent thinker, always challenging assumptions

- Smart and dedicated taskmaster, always looking for enabling technologies
- Contagiously optimistic, avoiding apostles of doom
- An innovator in changing times, breaking through comfort zones
- A mistake maker and risk taker, turning impossible dreams into results
- A visionary, finding opportunities within chaos
- A leader and coach, bringing forth the best in others

Additional behaviors that are desirable in a salesperson are listed as a sidebar on the next page. Conversely, if these behaviors are *not* in evidence, sales will suffer and targeted education is in order.

The rest of this section offers some other tips for education meant to fine-tune your sales approach.

Customer Survey

Consider a customer survey targeted toward learning how they respond to sales, and use this information to adjust your sales approach to best match your customers' attitudes. Select an adequate sampling from your current referral source base and ask a number of following questions. Revise your salespeople's selling approach based on the results.

- What do you like about salespeople?
- What don't you like about salespeople?
- What selling approach do you dislike?
- What is the best way for a salesperson to get your attention?
- What is the best way for a salesperson to get an appointment?
- What kind of voice-mail message would you return?
- How long do you typically spend with a salesperson?

BEHAVIORS OF SUCCESSFUL SALESPEOPLE

- Prospects aggressively for new customers
- Makes enough quality sales calls
- Follows through on commitments
- Asks ample probing questions
- Listens to the customer
- Determines and understands customer needs
- Plans every day, every sales call, and every presentation
- Convincingly explains the benefit-to-change to prospects
- Convincingly explains the benefit-*not*-to-change to customers
- Trial closes often enough
- Addresses objections before they arise
- Addresses the prospect's concerns head on
- Maintains a positive and contagious attitude
- Commits to self-improvement
- Sets and focuses on corporate and sales priorities
- Works smarter with enabling technologies
- Accepts accountability for responsibilities
- Turns customer relationships into client partnerships
- Adapts to and exploit change
- Manages time and resources
- Takes the initiative to be proactive
- Maintains the highest level of employee satisfaction
- Works your networks
- Meets and exceeds customer expectations
- Maintains high ethical standards

- When you receive a sales telephone call, what causes you to make an appointment?
- What is the best way to get you to move up a scheduled sales appointment?
- What do you expect from a salesperson during a sales call?

- Do you prefer a salesperson to have an appointment?
- When do you like to meet with salespeople?
- Do you really read the material salespeople leave?
- Do you have an example of what you think is an informative brochure?
- When you have a choice, why do you still refer to us?

In addition to a formal survey, your salespeople should informally get information from customers about your services and sales approach. When prospects agree to use your services, ask what convinced them to do so. Use their convictions to further fine-tune your selling approach.

Know What You Are Selling

Another facet of educating your sales force is to ensure that their sales techniques match what the prospect actually wants to purchase. Many healthcare providers sell their products and services without knowing what the consumer, customer, or end user is actually buying. Remember, people buy and refer for emotional satisfaction and then justify their decision with logic. You need to decide exactly what your customers are buying. They usually tie emotional satisfaction to safety, fear, greed, association, ego, and pride.

The After-"Yes" Sequence

After a prospect says "yes," he or she will refer or use your product or service. Consider having your salespeople execute the following new referral source sequence.

1. Thank the new referral source for the decision to refer verbally and in writing.

2. Reassure the new referral source that they made the right decision.
3. Ask the new referral source for a referral to a referral source.
4. Make a commitment to deliver something special, such as an article, additional information, etc..
5. Remind all the new referral sources' key office staff of the commitment to refer.
6. Ask when you can expect their first referral because you want to be present when their patient arrives.
7. Have your organization's senior person (if this is not you) call or write to thank the new referral source for their business and follow-up on all of the commitments made by your salespeople.
8. Provide your organization with the necessary information to make a great first impression.

The sidebar at the end of this chapter offers more tips you can incorporate into your efforts to educate your sales staff and give your organization a competitive edge. These tips address challenges that are unique to healthcare: selling to top executives and strategic account management. Also included is a selection of general tips for enhancing sales effectiveness.

Lost-Customer Analysis

Whenever business or customers are lost, assign a team to conduct an objective lost-customer analysis. Determine the root reason the business was lost, solve the problem, and then go after the lost business or customer.

COMMUNICATION

Keeping open communications with salespeople is critical to an organization's success. Employing one or more of the following resources enhances overall communication with salespeople.

- *Newsletter.* The newsletter should be a quick read and include enhancers and solutions to sales and selling scenarios, success stories, basic sales reinforcement, significant market trends, specific product information, progress reports, and key reminders. Using an electronic newsletter or faxed newsletter can save you time and money.
- *Electronic Q&A bulletin board.* Use the Internet to receive and answer questions from salespeople and customers.
- *Telephone Q&A bulletin board.* Use a telephone answering machine to receive input and questions from salespeople and customers.
- *Fax-on-demand services.* Arrange fax-on-demand services to both salespeople and customers, providing information about your products and services.
- *Audio tapes.* Use audio tapes to disseminate information to salespeople regarding product training, missed sales meetings, sales success stories, selling skills enhancement, progress reports, and new product introduction. Driving time is down time, so consider creating a down-time learning series.
- *E-mail.* Use e-mail to send significant and relevant information, personal progress reports, meeting information, updates, etc.

To be most effective, keep your communications simple, short, relevant, significant, and tied to increasing productivity, performance, and increasing incentives. Always be aware of the need to secure the information that is transmitted via wire, fiber, or air.

COMPENSATION

A sales compensation program attempts to differentiate pay within the sales force for results on the basis of accomplishing difficult, controllable sales tasks with consistency. Your approach to sales compensation should be a win-win scenario, in which the company and the salespeople achieve desired financial goals. The program should provide competitive compensation when results indicate that a high level of creative selling skills has been used to bring about desired results. Figures 8.5 and 8.6 are overviews of the most common sales compensation programs.

With a little gray-matter activity and a little trial and error, you should be able to create a sales compensation program that enforces self-motivation in salespeople, supports sales objectives, and stresses your organization's goals. The seven-step approach in Figure 8.7 can be used as a guide.

If a salesperson is not making a lot of money in salary and commission, then cash is the best way to motivate that person. However, if a salesperson is doing well financially, then noncash awards become the more powerful motivator. Use a diversity of cash, travel, and merchandise to recognize, reward, and motivate salespeople depending on their individual needs and wants. Refrain from changing the compensation program's core incentives without providing your salespeople appropriate notification and a sound business reason for doing so. Your top sellers (best paid) should be only those salespeople who best achieve corporate sales objectives. To reward consistent high performance without overcompensating salespeople who get lucky or bunch sales into one particular month, consider the following.

- Measure results for a high-performance compensation incentive over a period of three months or longer.
- Establish a minimum sales goal, whether based on dollar volume, gross revenue, full-line selling, etc., for the full period.
- Establish a monthly minimum that no single month can go below based on a percentage of your minimum sales goal.

FIGURE 8.5   SALES COMPENSATION PROGRAMS—SINGULAR PROGRAMS

Type	Influence Factor	Qualifications Factor	Appropriateness	Key Advantage	Key Distraction
Base Salary	Low	High	Market is mature and stable; established buying practices; multiyear contracts; strong base of repeat business; sales process is lengthy; and the Qualification Factor is high	Permits the company to stress training and team sales	No financial incentives to reinforce the company's sales objectives
Straight Com-mission	High	Low	Compensating nonemployee salespeople; emerging market or product line; weak competitive position; limited financial resources; short sales cycles; Influence Factor is high; and the selling process is highly focused on self-supervision and closing	Maximizes the incentive to succeed	The company sacrifices direction and control on the part of management

Influence Factor
An indicator of the relative importance of field sales in comparison with all other factors influencing the buying decision. If a company's advertising, promotions, and pricing are primarily responsible for its selling success, the field salesperson has a low influence factor. However, if the salesperson personally has to prospect, qualify, and influence the buyer to purchase a product or service, the salesperson has a high influence factor.

Qualification Factor
An indicator of the shortage of qualified individuals with the experience and/or educational background sufficient to meet the minimum industry selling skills re quirements.

At Risk
That portion of the compensation opportunity that is not guaranteed. Hence, "low risk" compensation is that portion of earnings (such as base salary) that the sales-person is virtually assured of receiving regardless of their productivity.

FIGURE 8.6   SALES COMPENSATION PROGRAMS—COMBINATION PROGRAMS

Type	Influence Factor	Qualifi-cations Factor	Appropriateness	Key Key Advantage	Key Key Distraction
Salary and Commission (Low Risk)	Low	x	Salespersons' influence factor is low, company products are recognized, and customer base is stable and loyal	Use of objective criteria to measure and reward differential sales performance, while maintaining the advantages of a base salary program	So much of the commission income is effectively assured that the actual percentage of pay truly at risk can become minuscule
Salary and Commission (High Risk)	High	High	Salespeople have considerable affect on short-term volume results, need to energize a mature sales force that is already receiving competitive base salaries, and both the Influence and Qualification Factors are high	Part or all of the base salary is treated as a guaranteed advance against incentive earnings	Competitors can lure salespeople by offering a larger and "low risk" base salary
Salary and Bonus	x	x	Sales cycle is long, volume is an incomplete indicator of sales effectiveness, account and product specific tasks and goals need reinforcement, the selling process is performed by a sales team, and the Influence and Qualification Factors are at neither extreme	The objective bonus is the most flexible form of sales incentive compensation; sales objectives can be translated into financial incentives	Subjectively determined bonuses have the obvious drawback of relying on after-the-fact judgment, which may not always be viewed as fair

Influence Factor
An indicator of the relative importance of field sales in comparison with all other factors influencing the buying decision. If a company's advertising, promotions, and pricing are primarily responsible for its selling success, the field salesperson has a low influence factor. However, if the salesperson personally has to prospect, qualify, and influence the buyer to purchase a product or service, the salesperson has a high influence factor.

Qualification Factor
An indicator of the shortage of qualified individuals with the experience and/or educational background sufficient to meet the minimum industry selling-skills requirements.

At Risk
That portion of the compensation opportunity that is not guaranteed. Hence, "low risk" compensation is that portion of earnings (such as base salary) that the salesperson is virtually assured of receiving regardless of their productivity.

FIGURE 8.7   PROCESS FOR DEVELOPING A SALES COMPENSATION PROGRAM

1. **Research**
   a. Know everything you can about your past sales and compensation programs—what worked and what did not work.
   b. Read one or more books on the subject (see references in the bibliography).
   c. Gather related industry specific data and information from industry associations and national suppliers.
2. **Define Objectives**
   a. List all your specific sales objectives based on corporate goals that a sales compensation program could help you accomplish.
   b. Consolidate sales objectives into several strategic objectives:
      1. increase gross revenue (from existing accounts);
      2. increase full-line sales revenue; and
      3. increase in new accounts.
3. **Determine Program Elements**. Determine the **type** of compensation program:
      1. base salary;
      2. straight commission;
      3. base salary—commission (low risk);
      4. base salary—commission (high risk); or
      5. combination program salary—bonus:
         a. the **target compensation** for different performance levels;
         b. the **results and activities** that will be rewarded; and
         c. the **pay formula** or rate at which you will pay for results.
4. **Test Program Parameters**
   a. Run your compensation program on a spreadsheet, testing various realistic scenarios.
   b. Evaluate the motivational impact or effect of the compensation program.
5. **Revise and Retest**. Fine-tune your program by revising it as needed.
6. **Create Final Sales Compensation Program Document**
   a. Finalize your draft into a finished compensation document.
   b. Ensure that the compensation program is easy to read and understand.
   c. Include example sales scenarios.
7. **Present Sales Compensation Program**. Start at the top and work down.

MOVING AHEAD

This section has offered an overview of an important and often overlooked aspect of healthcare marketing: sales. Yet all the clever marketing strategies and sales techniques in the world will not bring your organization success if the organization does not deliver on its promises and with every encounter give consumers a reason to be loyal. The following chapters explain how to provide customer service that will create loyalty among key customers.

TIPS FOR ENHANCING SALES EFFECTIVENESS: SELLING TO TOP EXECUTIVES

When selling to top executives, your salespeople need to:

- Know the names of their assistants and company's key players.
- Learn as much as possible about the company, its culture, its business, its industry, and its competition.
- Establish common ground with the top executive by showing a solid understanding of some key problems facing the company and/or its industry. Show how your organization can provide solutions and save them significant time and money.
- Avoid using your industry buzzwords, jargon, or technical mumbo jumbo. Speak in the prospect's tongue, using *their* buzzwords.
- Adhere to brevity. Do not waste the top executive's time; get to the point.
- Treat every "gatekeeper" (i.e., receptionist, assistant) with the same respect you would show the top executive. Make no exceptions. What goes around, comes around.
- Avoid insignificant conversation. Use an attention-getting opening that appeals to busy executives. Time is a premium; use it wisely.
- Involve the top executive by soliciting their opinion on something relevant to the industry.
- Listen for insights.
- Identify the specific goals, plans, and initiatives the top wants to achieve. Focus on the executive's focus.
- Inquire how the top executive selects his or her business partners. Ask who the company's best business partners are and why.
- Dress for success. Your attire should convey your (and your organization's) success.
- Ask for the business. Ask the top executive to give you the opportunity to save him or her time and money.

TIPS FOR ENHANCING SALES EFFECTIVENESS: STRATEGIC ACCOUNT MANAGEMENT

Today's healthcare organizations and health systems have many strategic accounts: managed care, employers, unions, business consortiums, regulators, and major referral sources and group practices. Take them seriously and treat them all like very important accounts that require management. Consider using the following account-management guidelines.

- Define your business objectives and priorities.

- Define your core product line and selling specialties.

- Profile and analyze current customers and prospects.

- Select your strategic accounts—those that will best enable you to achieve your business objectives.

- Create a strategic account-management structure: team members, team selling, team management, and account service and coordination.

- Select an executive for each strategic account team.

- Provide the necessary individual and team training for account responsibilities.

- Create information systems to support strategic account management.

- Create a performance-based compensation package for strategic account teams.

- Create a strategic account-management plan: account profiles, objectives, customer and prospect contact assignments, offered services, internal delivery coordination, research, follow-up, progress monitoring, and new business development.

- Coordinate communication channels and exchanges throughout your company—top to bottom, executive to staff, department to division.

- Search for new time- and money-saving solutions, partnership opportunities, and new product introductions with strategic accounts.

- Become a significant member of the strategic accounts troubleshooting team.

- Help your strategic account executives and personnel sell internally.

OTHER TIPS FOR ENHANCING SALES EFFECTIVENESS

Have your salespeople use one or more of the following to gain a competitive selling edge.

- Create an individual selling action plan for each prospect.
- Create individual referral source relationship-to-partnership plans.
- Create selling teams consisting of physicians, office managers and vendors.
- Create a list of reasons to visit a nonreferring referral source.
- Create a list of reasons to visit an existing referral source.
- Create a provider-of-choice image.
- Create a personal relationship-of-choice image.
- Send an attention-getting postcard.
- Send tubular mail.
- Send a full-size photograph introducing yourself.
- Send dynamic marketing collateral.
- Give a managed care chart.
- Speak at chamber, association, and society meetings.
- Write timely articles about your organization and its products and services.
- Be unique; elevate yourself above the me-too provider pool.
- Send a powerful letter of introduction announcing your intentions of calling for an appointment.
- Use colorful and unusual stamps on your correspondence.
- Use a three-minute timer to keep your telephone calls short.
- Use focus groups consisting of current referral sources to influence nonreferral sources.
- Conduct lunches with current and nonreferral sources to sell nonreferral sources.
- Ask your current referral sources why they refer; market their responses.
- Ask nonreferral source gatekeepers for help in getting their business.
- Make a service guarantee.

continued

OTHER TIPS FOR ENHANCING SALES EFFECTIVENESS *continued*

- Hold continuing education programs for both current and nonreferral sources.
- Engage in executive-to-executive meetings and lunches.
- Create physician-marketers to team sell.
- Use power names to gain appointments.
- Wear attention-getting buttons.
- Build your personal image by dressing for success.
- Enhance your presentation with relationship-building body language.
- Present a unique business card.
- Record your prospecting telephone conversations for later analysis (check local legality).
- Create a customized selling system and fine-tune it daily.
- Make a list of all the ways you can add value to your sales call.
- Be able to convincingly communicate benefit-to-change.
- Create and use attention-grabbing visual aids.
- Create promotional audio cassettes for your products and services.
- Use testimonials as direct-mail pieces.
- Start a web page.
- Join a local sales club.

SECTION THREE

Service

9

Mastering Customer Service

HEALTHCARE PROVIDERS HAVE many customer-related needs to address, including those of patients, referral sources, payers, employers, family members, and vendors. To provide superior service, every customer encounter and relationship needs to be dissected and analyzed from the customers' point of view. Only by examining each service element, as it contributes to lasting customer satisfaction, will you truly achieve the ultimate customer-friendly environment. A customer-friendly environment means your staff, operating policies, procedures, and protocols must be customer oriented. Remember that operating procedures that are convenient for your organization might not be satisfying for your customers. Work tirelessly with customers to improve the quality and delivery of your products and services. Your basic goals for customer service should be to:

- make it easy for customers to access or refer;
- be ready when customers do call or refer
- make it easy for customers to do business with you on a continuous basis; and
- thank customers for their patronage, trust, and referrals.

Satisfied customers are more likely to return to you and to refer others to you. Satisfied customers also minimize stress for staff, are less expensive to treat, and are less likely to sue. Most important, satisfied patients are easier to educate and more likely to follow their treatment regimen. Dissatisfied customers, on the other hand, do not return to your organization, and they may convey a negative impression of the organization to others. Dissatisfied customers increase stress for staff, are more expensive to treat, and are more likely to sue. Most important, dissatisfied patients are more difficult to educate and less likely to follow their treatment regimen.

The cost of dissatisfied customers may be higher than you think. I encourage healthcare executives to assess the cost associated with having a dissatisfied patient go through the system. Take into consideration all possible adverse events, medical procedures, or administrative scenarios. Your total cost estimate may be the catalyst for accelerating your quest for improved patient satisfaction. Share the information with every board member and employee. Patient satisfaction takes on a different perspective when you link lost dollars to it.

This chapter will help you understand your customers and what lies at the root of their satisfaction. It will offer a number of strategies for understanding the customer experience and improving your organization's processes to make them more customer friendly.

IDENTIFYING YOUR CUSTOMERS

Every organization needs to know who its customers are, both potential and current, internal and external. Even more important

LOSING YOUR PATIENTS MADE EASY

It takes five times more money to attract new customers than it does to retain existing ones. If you do not understand your patients, you will lose them. Losing patients is costly. Healthcare providers often lose their patients by:

- disregarding a patient's physical and mental discomfort.
- prolonging patient waiting time, especially without an explanation for the delay.
- being indifferent to your patients' problems and concerns. Inattention to customers by a member of your staff can cost your business between 15 and 30 percent of its gross revenue.
- compromising patient dignity before, during, and after examinations and procedures.
- breaching patient confidentiality.
- being insensitive when collecting payment.
- being rude in requesting patient insurance information and medical history.
- failing to effectively respond to a patient's communication needs and cultural differences.
- showing disrespect toward patient family members and guests.
- exposing your patients to an unsanitary or unsafe environment.
- treating your adult patients as children.
- misleading your patients about their medical condition.

Using these reasons as a starting point, begin every staff meeting with a five-minute discussion on improving customer service.

than senior management knowing the organization's customers, every employee in your organization needs to know who his or her customers are. Remember that customers can include patients, family members, members of the general public, vendors, community leaders, medical staff, and many others. Consider completing a customer analysis for each position within your organization, and make it a part of every job description. The customer analysis form in Figure 9.1 offers a good starting point.

FIGURE 9.1   CUSTOMER ANALYSIS FORM

	Customer Analysis				
Position: Main Telephone Operator					
	Encounter		Contact		Services Provided
Customer Type	Internal	External	Direct	Indirect	
Anyone calling into the hospital; visitors; and patients	–On telephone –In person	Call in on telephone	In person		–Welcome –Information –Directions –Assistance –Referral –Transfer call –Farewell
Medical Staff	–On telephone –In person	Call in on telephone	In person	Passed-on message accuracy	–Welcome –Information –Directions –Assistance –Referral –Transfer call –Messages –Farewell

UNDERSTANDING CUSTOMER SATISFACTION

Customer satisfaction is subjective. What makes one person happy might upset another. Just like quality, customer satisfaction is a personal perception about the quality of your products and services. What you believe is quality and satisfaction is of little value in the mind of the end user—the customer. A 1998 report by the Rhode Island Department of Health, "Quality Hospital Care: What Does It Mean?", supports the idea that consumers and providers have different perceptions of what constitutes quality care. The report found that consumers perceive quality care in terms of the treatment they receive, while providers view quality in terms of outcomes. The report states that although providers are aware of consumers' expectations, they believe that bureaucracy and paperwork prevent them from being more responsive to their patients by limiting the amount of time they spend with them.

Each customer forms his or her own short-term opinion (we will discuss long-term opinions later) based on the following perception factors.

- *Knowledge:* the customer's previous understanding about their needs and wants as they relate to your products, services, organization, personnel, etc.
- *Experience:* the customer's past experiences, both active and passive, with your organization and your competition. These experiences include those of certain third parties such as family members or friends.
- *Expectations:* the customer's perception of what to expect in doing business with you, based on matters such as previous knowledge, past experience, your advertising, consumer group articles, and third-party testimonials.

- *Reality:* the customer's firsthand service and staff encounters, the perceived value of medical intervention, treatment of family and friends, open and honest communications, payment process, and the total healthcare experience.

The customer's expectations and perceptions must become your reality, or you are not delivering ultimate customer satisfaction. Healthcare executives must always consider customer perception when trying to assess the quality of services.

THE LONG AND SHORT OF IT

Two segments comprise customer satisfaction: long-term and short-term satisfaction. When a patient leaves your facility satisfied, then initial treatment and service met the patient's short-term expectations. However, several weeks after returning home and discussing the incident with others, the patient's short-term satisfaction can turn into long-term dissatisfaction. For example, if the patient concludes that he or she paid too much, the patient's short-term satisfaction gives way to long-term dissatisfaction. A customer's satisfaction may start high but decline over time. The customer satisfaction flowchart in Figure 9.2 details the process. Organizations need to maximize both short-term and long-term satisfaction.

PREVAILING CUSTOMER DIFFERENCES ACROSS INDUSTRIES

According to the University of Michigan School of Business's American Customer Satisfaction Index (www.bus.umich.edu/research/nqrc/acsi.html), the following distinctions among customers are common across all industries and offer important strategic insight into customer satisfaction issues within healthcare.

FIGURE 9.2   TOTAL CUSTOMER SATISFACTION

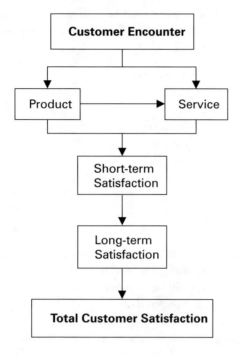

- Satisfaction rises with age, with the major increase in satisfaction among those age 55 and over
- Satisfaction declines as socioeconomic status rises for products and services of private companies
- Nonmetropolitan customers are more satisfied than those in metropolitan areas
- Differences in customer satisfaction among varying racial and ethnic groups are largely influenced by education levels
- Customer satisfaction is higher for manufactured goods than for services
- Customers are more satisfied with private sector services than with those provided by the government

MINDING YOUR Ps AND Qs

Perception is reality. When formulating an opinion about an organization's service, most customers consider one or more of the following personal perception factors:

Parking**	Procedure*
Place*	Pain*
Pleasantries*	Payment
Personnel*	Problems
Processing	Palatable*
Paperwork**	Prestige
Price**	Purpose
Physician*	Plan

* Pediatric focus

** Geriatric focus

Because patients cannot usually measure procedural appropriateness, technical expertise, or quality outcomes, they rely on personal experiences. Patients measure overall quality by easy access, feeling better, and low out-of-pocket costs.

Minding your Qs is a little more difficult. Prospects and consumers simply assume that you provide quality care and services, so you must deliver more. Pursue best quality and improve your quickness in responding to customer needs.

ULTIMATE CUSTOMER SATISFACTION

The key concept in customer satisfaction and service is continuity. Customers must be able to move from contact point to contact point smoothly without confusion, repetition, or interruption. One way of visualizing this concept is as a circle of trust. A patient's trust in the healthcare delivery system starts with his or her personal physician. That trust is then reinforced by the physician's office staff, passed along to the physician's hospital or other providers of choice, and referred to a specialist. The cycle ends with the initial physician. When it comes to patient satisfaction and loyalty, the circle of trust can have no dead ends.

Customer service can also be viewed as a relay race of satisfaction. A satisfaction relay starts with the preservice contact, passes through the service phase, and finishes with post-service follow-up. The customer is your baton, and, just like a baton, the customer can be dropped, potentially costing the organization hundreds of seconds in the race to win customer loyalty. For the most part, winning the customers' satisfaction is a team effort. Employees repeatedly run daily customer satisfaction races throughout an organization's life. Lose too many races and you lose it all—your customers and your longevity.

Customer service might also be viewed as a journey, but unlike most journeys that begin with the first step and end with the last step, the journey to ultimate customer service is never-ending. With every level of customer satisfaction you achieve, your customers will force you to move to a higher level as they grow to expect more.

By embracing these seven strategic steps, your organization will be well on its way in its journey toward achieving ultimate customer satisfaction.

1. *Determine* customers' interests, needs, perceptions, and wants.
2. *Define* those interests, needs, perceptions, and wants in terms of products and services.
3. *Develop* those products and services as defined by the customer.
4. *Deliver* the developed products and services from a customer's orientation and perspective.
5. *Delight* customers by exceeding their expectations whenever possible.
6. *Discover* new and better ways for delighting your customers with consistency.
7. *Dedicate* the necessary people, training, and resources to succeed.

These steps should create an organizational mindset that will never be satisfied with its customers' satisfaction. Your staff and operating procedures will be truly customer oriented. You will make every effort to become an indispensable part of your customers' interests, needs, perceptions, wants, or success, and you will constantly work with each customer to improve quality and personalize delivery of your products and services from their perspective.

ILLITERACY AND HEALTHCARE

Patient illiteracy often plays an adverse role in delivering healthcare services cost effectively. The patient's ability to be compliant, complete surveys, and follow directions affects their relationship with your facility. According to the Department of Education and Center for Health Care Strategies, Inc:

- 21 percent of adults, or 40 to 44 million people, are functionally illiterate, reading at or below a fifth-grade level.

- Another 25 percent of adults, about 50 million people, are marginally literate, meaning they cannot understand, interpret, and apply written material to accomplish daily tasks.

- More than 40 percent of chronically ill Americans are functionally illiterate.

- More than 66 percent of people older than 60 have inadequate literacy skills.

- Low literacy patients are 52 percent more likely to be hospitalized than those with adequate literacy skills.

Evaluate every written and visual communication your organization produces, and decide if they deliver your message to even the most literacy-challenged customer.

Sources: a. National Adult Literacy Survey and the Center for Health Care Strategies. 1993. U.S. Department of Education, Princeton University.
b. Parker et al. 1995. "The Test of Functional Health Literacy in Adults: A New Instrument For Measuring Patients' Literacy Skills." *Journal of General Internal Medicine* 10: 537–41.

SERVICE TRIAD

Many healthcare organizations forget that the total service event comprises three critical interlocking phases. Because they affect both short- and long-term satisfaction, ultimate customer satisfaction requires planning for all three of the service-triad phases.

1. *Pre*-service—connecting with a potential customer or patient
2. *Actual* service—delivering customer encounter experience
3. *Post*-service—disconnecting service encounter experience and follow-up

Most marketing people only occupy themselves with the actual phase. Your job is to ensure that all three phases are addressed.

SERVICE PATHWAYS

Like clinical pathways, a healthcare organization also has service pathways. Healthcare professionals map clinical pathways by defining the ideal activities and processes for a given treatment. The pathway identifies the various people involved in the treatment and the activities of each throughout the process. This process can be used for service pathways as well to map the ideal process and activities involved in customer encounters. Follow these steps to create service pathways:

1. Identify all customer contact points.
2. Identify staff positions encountered by customers.
3. Conduct encounter analyses, listing all encounter experiences and events.
4. Determine the best way to deliver and maintain each encounter.
5. Redefine, revise, and document each customer encounter, including policy, procedures, and protocols.

Consider the typical physician office visit. Figure 9.3 breaks that visit into 30 customer encounters, in order of occurrence.

FIGURE 9.3   CUSTOMER-ENCOUNTER STEPS IN A PHYSICIAN OFFICE VISIT

Step	Encounter
1	Patient is contacted prior to arrival
2	Information is collected
3	Information is provided
4	Patient arrives at facility
5	Patient finds a parking space
6	Patient arrives at facility entrance
7	Patient arrives at check-in area
8	Patient and escort are greeted
9	Patient insurance coverage is verified
10	Patient's medical history is collected
11	Patient registration is completed
12	Consent forms are signed
13	**Patient waiting**
14	Patient is called to examination room
15	Patient meets staff member(s)
16	Patient receives instructions; questions are answered
17	Patient is prepared or taken to dressing room
18	Patient is taken to procedure room
19	Patient meets physician(s) and/or technologist
20	Procedure is completed
21	Patient receives post-procedure instructions
22	Patient receives medication and/or prescription
23	Patient is taken back to dressing area
24	Patient is taken to checkout area
25	Copayments and/or deductibles are reconciled
26	Follow-up visit is scheduled
27	Patient is given option to complete satisfaction survey
28	Patient leaves facility
29	Patient receives post-visit follow-up call
30	Patient is surveyed again in four to six weeks

To create a service pathway, have a designated person or team analyze each event. Their ultimate job is to improve each event from the customer's perspective.

Notice customer-encounter experience Step 13: patient waiting. Contemporary healthcare customer service calls for "patient atriums" or "reflection areas," not "waiting rooms." There are many ways to improve and enhance service at this critical point. Of course, the ideal customer service pathway would interact with other attempts to map and improve processes, which would result in improving service so the customer does not have to wait to begin with.

The company that has mastered and capitalized on the art of waiting is Disney, Inc. During your next visit to a Disney theme park, keep track of your waiting time versus actual activity time. You will spend the overwhelming percentage of your time standing in line. You wait to enter, to ride, to eat, to relieve, to buy, to see the light parade, and to leave. Total time spent: about eight hours of waiting for an hour or two of true activity. Yet through creative thinking and implementation, Disney makes waiting as satisfying an experience as possible. Of course satisfying people already in a good frame of mind, excited about the day, and with plenty of money is much easier than satisfying patients who arrive at your facility with stress or apprehension, are anxious about what the day holds, and possess little money.

Start creating lists of internal and external customer contact points. Use Figure 9.3 as a reference. Outline critical patient points, encounters, and interface dynamics. Convene teams as necessary to brainstorm for improvements to the processes involved in customer encounters. Focus especially on those critical areas that possess one or more of the following characteristics:

- High traffic volume
- High unit price
- Repeat problems
- Long delivery times and waits

IMPROVED SERVICE WHEN PATIENTS MUST WAIT

- Ensure greeting by a proactive, attentive person radiating a friendly, welcoming smile
- Cluster furniture into group settings, not elbows to knee caps
- Provide an open-air receptionist and check-in area
- Avoid sliding glass windows that isolate staff from patients
- Reduce optical pollution by eliminating unprofessional signage and taped postings
- Place a water cooler in the patient waiting area
- Improve lighting for reading small print, forms, and other materials
- Announce any appointment delays without making the patient ask
- Post informative, yet passive, advertising about policies and procedures
- Preintroduce staff and physician by displaying their photographs on a wall
- Provide appropriate joke books, cartoons, etc., to help release stress and anxiety
- Provide desks with a telephone for making local calls
- Do not require patients to write their name and social security number for others to see
- Replace plastic chairs and artificial plants with more welcoming furnishings
- Remove spots caused by people using walls and windows as headrests

- Multiple and different customer-staff encounters
- Elderly and/or specially challenged customer base
- Staff, including medical staff, possesses poor communication skills
- Replacement parts on order
- Staff unfamiliar with procedure, product, and service

Any customer area that increases the tendency for producing stress or pain is a solid candidate for close review as a potential flash-over-point for customer dissatisfaction. Focus on capturing customer complaints at points of dissension. A customer critical-contact analysis worksheet is provided (Figure 9.4) to help you start taking the customer's pulse at critical customer-contact points.

ULTIMATE PATIENT SATISFACTION

Your most important customer is the patient. All others are subservient to the patient. Ask your employees, "Did you do anything significant yesterday that enhanced our customer service, benchmarked our quality, improved our profitability, or increased our competitiveness?" Use the following checklist to prompt your employees by asking if their actions:

- assisted a patient?
- assisted a patient's family member?
- enhanced physician relations?
- reduced operating costs?
- acquired new business?
- enhanced facility image?
- helped a fellow employee?
- solved a problem?

- caused a problem?
- increased their employability?
- assumed new responsibilities?
- were outside their job description?
- could have been done better?
- made someone feel better?
- kept someone else from doing his or her job?

MOVING AHEAD

With this review of the basics of customer satisfaction, we can move on to more specific dimensions of understanding and improving customer satisfaction. The next chapter offers an overview of the various methods by which you can measure customers' reactions to your services, along with further tips on how to analyze that information and take advantage of opportunities to improve your service.

FIGURE 9.4   CUSTOMER-CONTACT POINT ANALYSIS

Customer-Contact Point Analysis

Facility/Department:

Activity/Process:

Customer-Contact Points	Current Process/Procedure	Potential Problem(s)	Enhanced Process/Procedure	Responsibility	
				Accountability	

The Essence of
Satisfaction Surveys

CUSTOMERS AND PATIENTS are busy people; fewer and fewer are willing to complete yet another survey, questionnaire, or comment card. Those who do may not typify the target customer or patient group. However, you still need to survey customer and patient satisfaction as a way to change the way your organization does things. You need to discover how things are currently being done, so they can be done better to reflect your customers' interests and needs. If you are surveying your customers but not changing the organization, then you are wasting time and money.

SO WHAT AND WHO CARES?

Surprisingly, the vast majority of healthcare providers rate their patient satisfaction in the high 90th percentile. If you do have high satisfaction ratings, do not feel too comfortable. Many customers, patients, and their family members do not complete satisfaction surveys honestly because of illiteracy, aversion to consequences of whistle-blowing, lack of time, or, they simply have nonassertive personalities. Despite the shortcomings of the findings, more than a few people and organizations are, or will be, studying your patient-satisfaction scores closely, including:

- future patients;
- family members;
- managed care organizations;
- employers;
- friends and coworkers;
- accreditation agencies;
- federal and local regulatory agencies;
- consumer advocacy groups;
- patient support groups; and
- chat-room participants.

In time, patient satisfaction, based on multidimensional outcome indicators, will dominate decision making and become the major consideration for choosing a doctor, hospital, or any healthcare service. Care-ism will be forced to dominate capitalism.

SURVEYING INSTRUMENTS

Healthcare organizations have five survey instruments at their disposal, as shown in Table 10.1. A benchmarking patient satisfaction survey program will employ all five approaches to ensure maximum response and insight. I prefer proactive surveys that permit interaction with the dissatisfied customer in real time, not after the fact.

Knowing what to survey is more important than conducting a survey. Most healthcare provider-patient encounter opportunities can be broken down into three major phases: before, actual,

TABLE 10.1   SATISFACTION SURVEY INSTRUMENTS

Survey Instrument	Considerations and Comments	Dynamics
Written	Upon checkout Follow-up in four to six weeks Open-ended questions Include return and recommend factors Enhance response with offering Periodically used a third-party agency Option for patients to keep their 　　anonymity	Passive—reactive
Telephone	Third-party caller Caller's personality Personality of caller's voice Next day's follow-up call Use a script Call between 9:00 AM and 9:00 PM Five-minute maximum	Passive—reactive
Focus Group	Dissatisfied patients Use a script Facilitator's personality Neutral location Participation offering Third-party facilitator Keeping group participants' anonymity	Passive—reactive
Point of Service	Pre-office visit telephone call Check-in Waiting Procedure Checkout Patient advocates Hotlines	Active—proactive
Mystery Patient	Experienced third party Employee-friendly process Confidentiality Pre-office arrangements Written reports Suggested improvements Knowledgeable mystery patients	Active—proactive

and after. These phases are illustrated for a physician-office visit in Table 10.2. When surveying for patient satisfaction, remember all three phases of the encounter process.

PATIENT SATISFACTION SURVEY ANALYSIS AND ACTION

Many healthcare providers contract with a third-party survey company and receive reports comparing their ratings with others providers, both from a local and national perspective. However, it never hurts to periodically analyze the raw data yourself. Analyze your customer and patient satisfaction by various categories. Figure 10.1 shows one format for comparing satisfaction findings. Although this figure shows findings related to managed care plans, the same format can be used for comparing patient satisfaction among physicians or organization services.

As mentioned in the previous chapter, knowledge of opportunities to improve customer service must be acted on, especially to improve your processes related to customer service. The following process can be used once analysis of satisfaction data shows an opportunity for improvement.

TABLE 10.2   RANGE OF PATIENT ENCOUNTERS—PHYSICIAN PRACTICE

Pre-Office Visits	Actual Office Visits	Post-Office Visits
Schedule an office visit	Staff greeting	Diagnostic test results
Personal information	Verifying information	Schedule another visit
Medical history	Educating	Check patients' progress
Healthcare coverage	Reflective time (waiting)	Check patients' compliance
Payment method	Meet the physician	Refer to a specialist
Pre-office visit information	Medical intervention	Payment and collections
Procedure information	Instructions	Satisfaction surveys
Directions to office	Checkout	Thank you

FIGURE 10.1   PATIENT SATISFACTION COMPARISON—MANAGED CARE PLANS

Managed Care Plan	Very Satisfied	Satisfied	Dissatisfied	Very Dissatisfied	Total Surveyed	% Total Referrals
Blue Cross	350	796	3	1	1,150	79
United HC	85	1,334	23	44	1,486	93
USA	22	600	99	12	733	52
Health Choice	880	150	0	0	1,130	98
Totals	1,337	2,880	125	57	4,226	81

1. Set priorities among the identified opportunities for improvement. High priority should be placed on those that involve a large number of patients, that are traditionally problem-prone, that involve a large amount of money, or that can result in serious dissatisfaction.
2. Create teams of people involved with the process. Empower those teams to take action.
3. Analyze the process in detail. The team should use tools such as flowcharts and Pareto diagrams to understand how a process functions and which parts of the process are most likely to create customer dissatisfaction.
4. Recommend actions. The team should identify possible actions that will improve the process.
5. Test the actions. The modified or redesigned process should be implemented for a limited amount of time and data should be collected to determine whether the actions have had a positive effect.
6. Follow-up. If the changes are beneficial, make them part of standard operating procedures. If the changes are not helpful, recommend and test other changes. Revisit the process periodically to ensure that the improvements are sustained.

MYSTERY-PATIENT SERVICES

The "mystery-shopper" technique has long been used by the retail and restaurant industry as a check and balance system against the traditional customer questionnaire and telephone survey because it provides insight into how an organization is really delivering customer service. Mystery-patient services and surveys are a direct mystery shopper spinoff. If you want specific insight into how well your organization is delivering customer service, a mystery patient will provide a different, but very useful, perspective. Table 10.3 compares direct and mystery surveying. You should consider the following key points when setting up a mystery patient process.

- *Employee-friendly process.* All mystery patient activities need to be employee friendly, focusing on the customer's experience during their actual service encounter. Informing all employees up front that mystery-patient services are part of your total customer survey process is critical to success.
- *Knowledgeable mystery-patient surveyors.* Mystery-patient surveyors should be experienced in the following areas: healthcare, customer service and patient satisfaction dynamics, and mystery-patient surveying. Surveyors should know not only whether the service provided was good or bad, but what should have been delivered.
- *Detailed report.* Require a detailed written report. If possible, provide a video report for staff to play at meetings.
- *Recommendation to rectify areas of concern.* Besides pointing out areas of concern, a mystery-patient service should provide suggestions for improving those areas.
- *Ability to train employees.* Ideally, the mystery-patient service can provide related on-site training to augment current employee customer service and patient satisfaction programs, including areas of concern.

TABLE 10.3   MYSTERY SURVEY COMPARISON

	Direct Customer Survey	Mystery Patient Survey
Data extent	Organizational level (broad)	Activity level (specific)
Operational perspective	Strategic	Tactical
Survey reports	Customer's rerceptions (feelings)	Employees' performance (facts)
Data's appropriate usage	Reactive strategy and planning	Quick action
Orientation	Customer satisfaction	Customer service
Focus	Delivery experienced	Delivery process
Period	Remembered time	Real time

Mystery-patient surveys can also be important instruments for checking compliance with Medicare rules and regulations.

CUSTOMER COMPLAINTS WELCOMED

You *want* your customers and patients to complain because complaints are your barometer for measuring service levels. When expectations are not met, most patients simply go elsewhere without a single complaint. A complaint is a wake-up call, so take it seriously. Turn complaints into opportunities to show you really care. Patients and their family members complain most often because:

- the patient did not get what he or she expected.
- someone was rude to the patient.
- no staff member went out of his or her way to provide service.
- the patient experienced indifference from staff or did not believe he or she was being taken seriously.
- no one seemed to listen to the patient's questions or concerns.

- no one satisfactorily answered the patient's questions or addressed the concerns in a timely fashion.
- the patient encountered an employee with a negative attitude.
- the facility or the patient's room was dirty.
- someone embarrassed the patient.
- the patient was tired, under stress, or frustrated.
- the patient felt that an employee was not properly trained.
- the patient felt the lack of service was because an employee was prejudiced.

Any manager wanting to create a first-rate complaint system that starts showing results within six months should consider using the following five steps as their guide. Done right, your customer will start noticing positive changes within 30 days.

1. Issue a policy statement that says your organization embraces complaints. View complaints as opportunities.
2. Establish an implementation team with representatives from each step in the complaint-handling process, and identify each step in the process.
3. Establish a tracking system to record and classify complaints. The difference between your process and the best-in-business process is known as the gap. A gap analysis will show you what to improve.
4. Develop recommendations to improve your core processes and empower frontline employees to resolve complaints on first contact.
5. Put together an action plan for implementing the approved recommendations.

When establishing your staff's ability to deliver the highest patient-satisfaction level possible, be aware of third-party influences and account for any potential adverse effects such as:

- a patient's inpatient or outpatient status;
- admissions and discharge processes;
- patient-staff encounters;
- patient-physician encounters;
- billing and collection methodology;
- amenities and food;
- facility, parking, and safety; and
- ancillary support services.

Third-party influences may lower your overall customer and patient satisfaction. You will benefit by using mystery-patient services to assess third-party providers and collect competitor intelligence.

CREATING A DISSATISFIED-PATIENT PROFILE

Creating dissatisfied-patient profiles greatly helps an organization identify its potentially dissatisfied patients, sometimes even before the patient arrives. Collect as much of the following information for all patients before their arrival, and convert them into a dissatisfied-patient profile.

- Age
- Marital status
- Education
- Procedure
- Referral source
- Income level
- Healthcare coverage
- Payment method
- Staff encounter(s)
- Time of encounter
- Occupation
- Employer

Analyze your dissatisfied patient data, looking for common characteristics—the more found, the more accurate the profile. Create your dissatisfied-patient profile by correlating the data. Consider doing so for the organization as a whole, by department, and by physician. Using the statistically dissatisfied-patient-representative profile, identifying potentially dissatisfied patients is easier. The organization now can address the situation according to established policy dealing with dissatisfied patients. Before patients of a profile known to be dissatisfied are seen by your organization, you can contact the patient at home. Your staff can defuse the situation before it occurs, usually by creating realistic patient expectations and providing appropriate education. Keeping patients informed along the way is a sure way to keep them satisfied.

MOVING AHEAD

Of course customer service is more than just measuring patients' reactions and making improvements based on that information. You need to design high-quality customer service into your organization. One way to do that is to hire people who are enthusiastic about your customers and who display a passion for excellent service. The next chapter explains how to make sure your workforce is filled with people whose attitudes will translate into satisfied customers.

Attitude and Service

11

AN ATTITUDE OF dedication, enthusiasm, and consistency is paramount if you are going to provide superior customer service. Sometimes this service attitude is called "internal marketing." This chapter explores some methods for creating the right internal attitude for excellent customer service.

INTERVIEWING FOR ATTITUDE

During the interviewing process, keep your questions focused on past behavior that highlighted the candidate's attitude as it relates to customer service. It helps to define or profile the key attitude traits you desire in employees. Consider using some of the following screening questions when interviewing potential new employees.

Judgment
- Tell me about the last time you broke the rules to serve a customer in need.
- Tell me about the last time you bent company policy to resolve a customer complaint.

Flexibility
- Tell me about the last time you compromised your position to make a customer happy.
- Tell me about the last time you took a different approach to solve a recurring customer problem.

Team Orientation
- Tell me about the last time you worked with others to successfully solve a critical problem.
- Tell me about the last time that you had to get others to actively participate in a specific team activity and what approach you took.

Unselfishness
- Tell me about the last time you did a great job but received no recognition.
- Tell me about the most significant sacrifice you made to fulfill a customer's need.
- Tell me about the most significant sacrifice you made to fulfill a company or coworker's need.

Humor
- Tell me about the last time you used humor to calm an upset coworker.
- Tell me about the last time you used humor to diffuse a tense customer situation.

Adaptability
- Tell me specifically how you have worked out a conflict with a difficult coworker.
- Tell me about the last time you had to create a policy on the spot to resolve a customer issue.

Courage

- Tell me about the last time you spoke out to change company policy for the betterment of customers.
- Tell me about the last time you made a serious mistake dealing with a customer and how the situation was rectified.
- Tell me about the last time you challenged a coworker whose performance was hurting customer service.

Service Orientation

- Tell me how you have contributed to improving customer service.
- Tell me about the last customer you helped who was not your direct responsibility.

Willingness to Learn

- Tell me about the most important career skill you learned in the last six months.
- Tell me about the last time you taught yourself a new skill and what motivated you to do so.

Risk Orientation

- Tell me about the last time you tried something new to improve customer service.
- Tell me about the last time you stuck your neck out to help another department, coworker, or customer.

Sacrifice

- Tell me about the last significant personal sacrifice you made to respond to a customer situation.
- Tell me about the last significant personal sacrifice you made to improve company performance and productivity.

Self-Improvement

- Tell me about the last successful effort you made toward self-improvement.
- Tell me about the last time you asked someone for help because you were not sure what to do next.

THE ROTTEN APPLE SYNDROME

When organizations tolerate attitude-challenged employees, managers, board members, or physicians, it is no different than throwing rotten apples in with the good—soon, they spoil the whole lot. So why are attitude-challenged people sometimes tolerated in healthcare? Many reasons exist:

- legal protection under various federal and state laws;
- nonassertive managers and supervisors;
- the employee's exclusive technical expertise;
- favoritism or nepotism;
- inadequate documentation to support dismissal;
- person's investment in the business; or
- performance (e.g., top-referring physician).

The above list is far from inclusive, and there are as many reasons for bad attitudes as there are people with bad attitudes. However, any attitude-challenged person can safely and legally be terminated with a little foresight, appropriately documented performance expectations related to attitude, and employee-awareness warnings.

ATTITUDE EXPECTATIONS

Every employee's job description should have one or more expectations related to attitude and customer service. These can help identify expectations for new staff, keep all staff focused on customer service and a positive attitude, and provide rationale for disciplinary action, if necessary.

Consider including at least one of the following types of statements in your employees' job descriptions.

- *Attitude statement.* Define the attitude needed. I call this "Great Expectations." Give employees a list of acceptable and unacceptable behavior. Have all employees sign the statement and place it in their personnel files so that it is understood up front that unacceptable behavior is grounds for termination. This is not legal advice but a common-sense suggestion.

- *Service statement.* Refer to customer service standards in all job descriptions. Define job-specific responsibilities and accountabilities for delivering customer and employee satisfaction.
- *Team statement.* Define the job's team participation, responsibilities, and requirements. Provide a list of potential teams.

Consider including one or more of the following specific performance expectations related to service in everyone's job description.

- You are responsible for creating and maintaining a customer satisfaction level that generates no more than _____ complaints, adverse issues, and negative situations per _____.

- You are responsible for promoting corporate philosophies; generating team spirit; and creating and maintaining a business environment that fosters employee satisfaction, maximum productivity, and profitability.
- You are responsible for adhering to, in good faith and spirit, our defined "Great Expectations" of acceptable and unacceptable behaviors.
- You are responsible for prioritizing your every thought, word, and action in the following order of business: customer first, company second, coworkers third, and you last.

Challenge your employees to come up with their own ways to better do their jobs, and treat them as volunteers, not employees.

EMPLOYEE SATISFACTION

Employee satisfaction is fundamental to customer satisfaction. Without satisfied employees, no healthcare organization or medical practice will deliver customer service at the level and consistency necessary to maintain leadership and dominate the competition position. This self-assessment should help senior executives determine to what extent they foster employee satisfaction. The survey can be adapted to be given to staff as well.

1. Does executive and senior management value employee satisfaction?
   ☐ Yes   ☐ Sometimes   ☐ No

2. Does our organization consistently promote employee relations?
   ☐ Yes   ☐ Sometimes   ☐ No

3. Do employees hear about important news through the grapevine or in the news media before hearing it from executive and senior management?
   ☐ Yes   ☐ Sometimes   ☐ No

4. Are our line managers and supervisors effective communicators?
   ☐ Yes   ☐ Sometimes   ☐ No

5. Does our organization provide line managers and supervisors with communications training?
   ☐ Yes   ☐ Sometimes   ☐ No

6. If your answer to #5 is yes, does the communications training stress both employee satisfaction and relationship building?
   ☐ Yes   ☐ Sometimes   ☐ No

7. How often does executive and senior management walk the corridors and visit departments to observe, listen, and learn employee concerns?
   ☐ Never   ☐ Sometimes   ☐ Always

8. How often does executive and senior management eat in the employee cafeteria to listen, learn, and discuss employee concerns?
   ☐ Never   ☐ Sometimes   ☐ Always

continued

EMPLOYEE SATISFACTION *continued*

9. How often does executive and senior management meet in informal meetings to listen, learn, and discuss employee concerns?

☐ Never ☐ Sometimes ☐ Always

10. When major organizational changes occur, are all employees included in the decision process?

☐ Yes ☐ Sometimes ☐ No

11. When major department changes occur, are its employees included in the decision process?

☐ Yes ☐ Sometimes ☐ No

12. Does our organization protect an employee's anonymity when the employee so wants?

☐ Yes ☐ Sometimes ☐ No

13. Does our organization conduct an employee-satisfaction survey?

☐ Yes ☐ Sometimes ☐ No

14. If your answer to #14 is yes, does our organization conduct its employee-satisfaction surveys at least annually?

☐ Yes ☐ Sometimes ☐ No

15. Does executive and senior management take the employee-satisfaction survey results seriously?

☐ Yes ☐ Sometimes ☐ No

16. Does executive and senior management openly discuss the survey results with employees?

☐ Yes ☐ Sometimes ☐ No

17. Based on survey results, does executive and senior management create a formal employee-satisfaction action plan?

☐ Yes ☐ Sometimes ☐ No

18. Is the employee-satisfaction action plan shared with all employees?

☐ Yes ☐ Sometimes ☐ No

continued

EMPLOYEE SATISFACTION *continued*

---

19. Does executive and senior management effectively follow-up with action plan items?
    ☐ Yes   ☐ Sometimes   ☐ No

20. Does executive and senior management convey action plan progress with all employees?
    ☐ Yes   ☐ Sometimes   ☐ No

21. Do our organization's employees feel appreciated?
    ☐ Yes   ☐ Sometimes   ☐ No

22. Do our organization's employees believe they can make a difference on how we treat our customers?
    ☐ Yes   ☐ Sometimes   ☐ No

23. Do our organization's employees believe we empower them to resolve dissatisfied customer issues?
    ☐ Yes   ☐ Sometimes   ☐ No

If you answered "yes" or "always" to all 23 questions, your organization is a leader in employee relations. However, anything less shows the need to improve your organization's employee-relation efforts.

EVALUATIONS

Research shows that most personnel evaluations are subjective in nature. People whom evaluators like receive better evaluations than those less liked. I recommend objectivity when evaluating people. Only substantial performance outside of one's job description—saving the organization significant time and money or increasing revenue—warrants anything higher than a satisfactory rating. Excellent means consistently doing something significant toward corporate success. Further, and more important, those individuals achieving outstanding performance evaluations need outstanding rewards.

LEADERSHIP PRINCIPLES

Let us not forget how you as a healthcare executive contribute or detract from the scheme of things. Enhancing your leadership prowess is easy if you abide by the following guidelines:

- Be professional and proficient
- Know yourself and seek self-improvement
- Know your employees and look out for their welfare
- Keep your employees well informed
- Set the example for employees to emulate
- Ensure that tasks are understood, supervised, and accomplished
- Train your employees as a team
- Make sound and timely decisions, especially when employees are affected
- Develop a sense of responsibility among your employees
- Use your employees in accordance with their abilities
- Seek responsibility, fulfill obligations, and be accountable for your actions
- Be a good follower
- Have the courage to do right and to adhere to a higher standard of personal conduct
- Have the fortitude to make tough decisions under stress and pressure
- Do not bow to narcissism and nepotism

It is possible to divide leaders into two categories: those who do little but take most of the credit, and those who do most of the work and take little credit. Focus on being the latter; the competition is not as great.

THE TWELVE CEO COMMANDMENTS

The key to being a successful and effective CEO can be found in the three letters of CEO. Consider **E**xecuting your **O**ffice guided by the twelve CEO Commandments. The rest is success.

1. **C**ommunicate **E**ffectively with **O**thers.
2. **C**onstantly **E**xplore for **O**pportunities.
3. **C**hange to **E**xploit **O**pportunities.
4. **C**hannel **E**nergies to **O**bjectives.
5. **C**oach **E**mployees in **O**rganization.
6. **C**onvey **E**nergizing **O**ptimism.
7. **C**apitalize on **E**fficient **O**perations.
8. **C**onsolidate **E**fforts in **O**rganization.
9. **C**ut **E**xcesses from **O**rganization.
10. **C**ultivate **E**xcellence in **O**rganization.
11. **C**reate **E**xpertise in **O**rganization.
12. **C**urtail **E**xecutive **O**pulence.

In a nutshell, being an effective corporate coach is all about **C**ommunicating, **E**xecuting, and **O**ptimizing, in that order.

MOVING AHEAD

This section has delved into the many activities involved in hiring people, designing processes, and improving processes to ensure the optimal customer experience. In closing, I stress that healthcare marketing, sales, and service are nothing without the patient. If the patient is taken out of the healthcare mix, then all that is cared about is profit. "Care-ism" must always precede capitalism.

To this end, I have provided the following two appendices. Appendix A, National Patient Recognition Week, describes a week dedicated to recognizing and celebrating the reason for your professional existence: your patients.

Appendix B, Employee Training, explores insights into identifying training needs and how best to educate your employee base to better serve your patients.

Appendix A:
National Patient Recognition Week

National Patient Recognition Week is the first week in February, and National Patient Recognition Day is February 3rd. Those dates are set aside each year as a special time of patient recognition by all healthcare providers, patient services, and ancillary support personnel. Your organization should use this time to seriously reflect on your stewardship of patient care, your dedication to patient safety, and your commitment to patient satisfaction. National Patient Recognition Week and Day (NPRW and D) are special occasions for all people working in healthcare to reconfirm and demonstrate their renewed commitment to their field. We must all put care-ism before capitalism, lest we forget our reason for being. The following action items will help you and your organization reenergize the human side of patient care.

PHYSICIANS

Personal minute	Spend an extra personal minute with each patient to learn more about them and for them to learn more about you.
Positive body language	Spend the time to learn and use positive body language to reinforce your caring.

Personal thank you	Spend the time to thank your patients for choosing you as their doctor and for exhibiting confidence in your judgment and care.
Good patient kudos	Spend the time to recognize a good patient.
Hand holding	Spend more time making reassuring physical contact with your patients, especially those in the hospital.
Patient's shoes	Spend some time walking in your patients' shoes by sitting in an emergency department for an hour, eating lunch with a patient in their hospital room, or becoming a mystery patient yourself.
Explain more	Spend more time explaining what you are doing and why and reviewing all possible side effects and treatment options.
Start asking	Spend more time asking the patient what they think about you, your staff, their course of treatment, where they want to be referred, and their level of satisfaction.
Office activities	Spend some money for a special floral arrangement dedicated to patients; offer snacks, beverages, and treats; validate parking tickets; or have the office staff give each patient a coffee cup or a thank-you card with everyone's signature on it. Give each patient a tour of your office area, provide free health screening, and have your staff introduce themselves to patients and their family escorts. And smile more!

HOSPITALS

Patient Recognition Week

- Present a Medicare seminar for interested patients.
- Adopt a patient, ensuring special attention to the patient during their stay.
- Inaugurate a new patient service.
- Publish a special patient newsletter.
- Have a testimonial day: Convert patient testimonials into posters for display.
- Use a special meal tray placemat.
- Sponsor a thank-you poster contest for schools, staff, and departments.
- Create special moments of caring (extra smiles and more miles).
- Provide patient snack areas.
- Award good-patient certificates.
- Print thank-you tents for cafeteria table.
- Offer free classes for learning how to interpret/understand hospital and medical bills.
- Suggest that executives and managers eat lunch with patients.
- Spend an extra hour of your time with a patient each day.
- Have employees go through admission process, wait in the emergency department, or become a volunteer.
- Develop interactive patient social events at floor level or systemwide.
- Initiate special health screenings.
- Decorate a patient waiting area or relaxation room.
- Provide free mammograms within the recommended guidelines.
- Offer special day and evening healthcare educational classes.
- Have management and staff sign a pledge or statement to excel at patient satisfaction.

- Open and dedicate an Internet healthcare information workstation for patients and families.
- Send patients get-well cards signed by attending staff and/or administrator.
- Work with local radio, television, and news reporters to create awareness.

Patient Recognition Day

- Express your appreciation by offering free:
  — parking for patient and visitors;
  — cafeteria purchases within specified limits;
  — coffee and donuts in morning;
  — promotional T-shirts;
  — newspapers; and
  — videos/movies.
- Dedicate a special patient inner-peace sanctuary or garden.
- Put flowers in patient rooms.
- Offer gift shop discounts.
- Make a special dessert.
- Throw a recognition party for all patients (come as you are).
- Have management assume volunteer positions for day.
- Create a special recognition program for patients and family members.
- Recognize your oldest and youngest patient.
- Have executives, managers, and employees give up an hour or day's pay to help a needy patient.
- Plant a tree of recognition.
- Conduct hospital tours.
- Have the administrator or CEO take discharged patients to their waiting transportation.
- Have the administrator or CEO personally thank every patient for using their facility.
- Create a special patient coffee mug, certificate, goodie bag, magnet, balloon, or sticker.

- Get to know more about your patients by visiting with them longer and on your own time.
- Read the newspaper or a book to those patients that cannot read for themselves.
- Design and dedicate a patient web site.
- Change computer screen savers to a patient satisfaction reminder.
- E-mail a patient-satisfaction reminder to staff.
- Make a New Year's resolution about patient satisfaction.
- Assign patients a private room when admitted on February 3rd.

ORGANIZATION/PRIVATE GROUP PRACTICE

- Begin every meeting with a patient recognition statement.
- Start a patient-recognition think tank to plan for this special occasion.
- Offer cultural awareness and sensitivity classes for employees.
- Start an essay contest, "Why I care about my patients."
- Review patient rights with every employee and at new employee orientations.
- Provide easy access for patients to voice a complaint by telephone, in writing, and in person.
- Distribute patient-care ribbons, badge of caring, etc.
- Create an oath of care, then live and reward by it.
- Distribute customer-service and patient-satisfaction materials to every employee.
- Send out patient thank-you cards.
- Role play employee-patient encounter situations using good and bad scenarios.
- Clean up your coding and billing errors.
- Be a proactive patient advocate.

NPRW PROCLAMATION

Consider contacting your state's governor and having an official NPRW and D proclamation issued and signed. Be the first in your state to do so and use the coattail publicity to your advantage. The public relations factor is great for all concerned parties. Solicit city officials, senators, and even the White House. As an example, Alabama's Governor Don Siegelman signed such an NPRW proclamation on January 7, 2000 to become one of the progressive states undertaking this historical event for all patients.

I hope that by participating in National Patient Recognition Week, healthcare providers will reinforce their commitment to patient care. In the process, they will form caring habits that will live on in each of us.

Appendix B:
Employee Training

The successful executive-coach knows that employee training is important to all facets of customer service and other on-the-job activities, and acts accordingly. Knowledge is power, and it is a wise company that strives to educate its employee base. The training process shown in Table A.1 highlights how to maximize training efforts.

IMPROVING TEAM PRODUCTIVITY

The bigger the healthcare entity, the better a team can excel. Executive-coaches know this and work to maximize the organization's team productivity:

> **T**ogether **E**veryone **A**chieves **M**ore

for all and all for the patient's well-being. Getting your teams' productivity up and running on all cylinders is easy. Comply with the team productivity steps in Table A.2, and your teams will perform beyond your expectations. Teams are only as good as their executive support.

TABLE A.1 TRAINING PROCESS

Basics	Principles	Elements	Reinforcement
Tell the person how	Present meaningful information, minimize the fluff	Team leader must have both knowledge and experience in the subject	Refresher courses
Show the person how	Present only one idea or concept at a time	People must be motivated to pay attention	Progress journals and daily activity logs
Let the person practice what they have learned	Present information in a way that is easily comprehended and mastered	Use plain, intelligent, and understandable English	Training and performance aids
Ensure the person is doing it correctly	Present frequent summaries and get feedback to ensure understanding	New information and material must be associated to something with which the person is already familiar	Follow-up activities, testing, and performance reviews
		The best learning process challenges people to study for themselves	Failure analysis
		Make material applicable to the job	Positive reinforcement

TABLE A.2   TEAM PRODUCTIVITY

Step	Action
1. **Define**	Defining the team's goals and each team member's objectives, expectations, and performance levels.
2. **Determine**	Determining the availability and allocation of resources, critical dates, and workflow.
3. **Delegate**	Delegating appropriate empowerment, responsibility, and accountability to each team member.
4. **Deregulate**	Deregulating working constraints, freeing the spirit and mind, focusing on objectives and achievements, and rewarding success.
5. **Dedication**	Dedicating the necessary time, resources, and management support to achieve assigned team goals, especially on a personal basis.
6. **Dissolve**	Dissolving disruptive internal and external conflict in a timely fashion, providing the team leader with the authority and support to act accordingly.
7. **Demonstrate**	Demonstrating a sense of importance in achieving the team's goals and individual member's personal worth to the team effort.

THE ART OF TEACHING ADULTS

The key points of many adult training programs are highlighted in the following four tables. Basically, adult learners have three primary reasons for pursuing learning. Table A.3 outlines the major characteristics of these three learner types. Most healthcare, medical, and professional continuing education is goal focused, concentrating on licensing, certification, new equipment, and job related self improvement.

TABLE A.3 ADULT LEARNER TYPES

Goal Focused	Activity Focused	Learner Focused
Knowledge must be put to immediate use personally or professionally	Pursue education for reasons having no connection with either the content or the purpose of the training	They seek knowledge for the sake of knowledge or out of the desire to know
Pursuit of a purpose or sharply defined goal/objective(s) is the primary motivation for education	In many instances, they use education as an escape	Possess a continuity and range of experiences that make participation more than the sum of its parts
Much of the education is episodic in nature; however, the episodes are a never ending part of their life	They are often in need of some socioemotional fulfillment such as peer recognition	Typically, they are avid readers
They seek immediate satisfaction when an educational need or interest appears	Often seek nothing more than socializing	Education is best described as constant, rather than continuing, to their learning
The purpose always initiates the educational effort	Some pursue education to compile credits, certification, and diplomas	What they do allows a continuous flow and continuity to their lifetime learning
	They are the proverbial student	
	In many cases, the competition of activity and the fulfillment it brings is important in and of itself	

ADULT LEARNING DYNAMICS

The adult learning dynamics table (Table A.4) shows the various relationships between the teaching approach (medium), highly technical and low-technical information, and the key sensory learning elements. Notice that a kinesthetic teaching approach is best for highly technical information, dexterity, and skills (e.g., organ transplants). However, when conducting low-tech training, the visual approach works best (e.g., learning a new software program). Use the information contained within this book as a thinking catalyst or a mental springboard. Case studies often become the traditional box we find ourselves trapped within. The triad of innovation, motivation, and perspiration is what one needs to succeed.

TABLE A.4   ADULT LEARNING DYNAMICS

Medium	High Tech (hard)	Low Tech (soft)	Key Sensory Learning Elements
Audio	10%	35%	Ears (sound, voice, inflection, tone)
Visual	25%	**50%**	Eyes (animation, color, relationships)
Kinesthetic	**65%**	15%	Multiple senses (ears, eyes, hands, feet)
Focus	Do it (hands) Technical-detailed case studies **66%**	See it (mind) Conceptional Role playing 33%	Activity orientation Subject and material complexity Analytical methodology important Segmentation of adult population

POST-TRAINING EVALUATION

After completing a training session, post-training evaluation is the next step. During this phase, you need to reinforce the training, evaluate performance enhancement levels, and measure the return on investment. Consider implementing the post-training evaluation format shown in Table A.5.

TABLE A.5   POST-TRAINING EVALUATION

Activity	Weeks	Person	Comments
Reinforcement	1	Trainee	Everyday for six to seven days to enhance retention
Evaluation	3–4	Supervisor	Real-time performance evaluation
Post Training Benefits	10–12	Supervisor/ Financial	Long-term performance improvement versus training investment

INFORMATION EXCHANGE

Best teaching practices focus on positive transfer learning. Negative transfer approaches make the process of learning and retention difficult. Table A.6 compares the key elements of information transfer.

TABLE A.6   INFORMATION EXCHANGE

	Key Elements	Positive Transfer	Negative Transfer
Conceptions	Previous awareness or experience with the information and processes	Familiar (experienced)	Unfamiliar (new)
"Reliability"	Can relate to the information and processes	Linking	Disassociating
Transferability	Can grasp the new information and processes	Maximum	Minimum
Experience	Total learning process	Supportive	Intimidating

The total managed care experience—deep discounting, curtailed decision making, quality standards, practice guidelines, controlled referrals, reengineering, and patient satisfaction—can be difficult for healthcare providers to learn. The managed care information exchange is more of a negative transfer than a positive one. However, by approaching the whole process from a different perspective, the healthcare industry can begin a self-imposed and self-administrated reform process.

IDENTIFYING TRAINING NEEDS AND REQUIREMENTS

The first golden rule of training is to know who, what, why, where, when, and how you are training. The second golden rule is to expect results. The training needs-assessment worksheet shown in Figure A.1 is easy to reconstruct and complete. Use it as a guide to determine the results your key players expect from the training program.

To maximize an organization's training time and dollars, all training—budgeted or otherwise—needs submission with similar justification.

FIGURE A.1   TRAINING NEEDS ASSESSMENT

Determine	Trainee	Supervisor	Top Executive	Customer
Who				
What				
Why				
When				
Where				
How				
Desired Results				
performance				
investment				

Information Resources

THIS RESOURCE REFERENCE lists publications, products, and sources from a variety of manufacturers, publishers, and suppliers that can help your marketing and sales goals.

RESEARCH DATA AND INFORMATION

Acute Low Back Problems in Adults published by the Agency for Healthcare Research and Quality (800/358–9295)

American Demographics Magazine available from Intertec Publishing (800/828–1133)

American Medical Association catalog of products (800/621–8335)

Case Management Resource Guide published by Dorland Healthcare Information (800/627–2244)

Chamber of Commerce (local)

Congressional Research Service Reports (contact your congressional representative)

Dartmouth Atlas of Healthcare available through the American Hospital Association (800/242–2626)

Healthcare Almanac Yearbook published by Thompson Financial Media (800/535–8403)

Healthcare Market Reporter newsletter from the Managed Care Information Center (800/516–4343)

Health, United States printed by the United States Government Printing Office (202/512–1800)

Joint Commission on Accreditation of Healthcare Organizations, JCAHO (630/792–5000)

Journal of Interactive Marketing published by John Wiley & Sons (212/ 850–6645)

Libraries designated as repositories of federal publications

Medicare Cost Reports (Freedom of Information Act)

Mental Health, United States printed by United States Government Printing Office (202/512–1800)

Modern Healthcare Daily FAX from Crane Communications (800/678–9595)

National Center for Health Statistics (301/458–4636)

National Health Care Anti-Fraud Association (202/659–5955)

People's Medical Society (800/624–8773)

Public Citizen (202/588–1000)

Psychology and Marketing published by John Wiley & Sons (212/ 850–6645)

State medical and professional associations

State Insurance Commission

State Hospital Association

State health planning and regulatory agencies

State Self-Insured Employer Association

St. Lucie Press, book catalog (800/272–7737)

MANAGED CARE BOOKS, NEWSLETTERS, AND INFORMATION

American Association of Health Plans (202/778–3247)

American College of Healthcare Executives/Health Administration Press, publication catalog (301/362–6905)

Business & Health published by Medical Economics, Inc. (800/ 432–4570)

Capital Publications, Inc./Aspen Publishers (800/655–5597)

Health Insurance Associates of America (800/848–0773)

HMO-PPO Digest published by The Business Word (800/529–9615)

HMO/PPO Directory from Medical Economics, Inc. (800/222–3045)

HMO Industry Profile (202/778–3247)

Managed Care Local Market Overview published by Dorland Healthcare Information (800/627–2244)

Managed Care Facts, Trends and Data, and the *Managed Care Week* newsletter published by Atlantic Information Services, Inc. (800/521–4323)

The Managed Care Year Book and *The Executive Report on Managed Care* from Health Resources Publishing/Managed Care Information Center (800/516–4343)

National Committee for Quality Assurance Health Plan Report Card (800/839–6487) www.ncqa.org

MANAGED CARE CONTRACTING

Healthcare Capitation & Risk Contracting Manual published by Thompson Publishing Group (800/934–1610)

HMO-PPO Databases published by Dorland Healthcare Information (800/627–2244)

Main Street Software (800/548–2256)

SALES CONTACT MANAGEMENT SOFTWARE

Act! www.actsoftware.com

Telemagic www.telemagic.com

SALES AND SALES MANAGEMENT

Boardroom Reports Publisher (800/234–3834)

Dartnell Corporation (800/621–5463)

Executive Book Summaries (800/521–1227)
McGraw-Hill/Health Professions Division (800/634–3966)
National Association of Sales Professionals (800/489–3435)
Sales and Marketing Management (800/821–6897)
Selling Power (800/752–7355)

BUSINESS AND MARKETING PRODUCTS AND SOFTWARE

Inc. (800/468–0800)
Office Depot, Office Max, and CompUSA retail stores

DATABASE SOFTWARE

Alpha Five (800/451–1018) www.alphasoftware.com
Lotus Approach (800/343–5414) www.lotus.com
Microsoft Access (800/426–9400) www.microsoft.com/access

MAPPING SOFTWARE

MapLink (800/370–8967)

BROCHURE MATERIALS AND SOFTWARE

Beaver Prints (814/742–6070) www.beaverprints.com
My Brochures, Mailers, and More (800/325–3508)
Paper Direct products and software (800/272–7377) www.paper-direct.com

HEALTHCARE ONLINE

The Online Guide to Healthcare Management and Medicine
    McGraw-Hill/Health Professions Division (800/634–3966)
The Online Consumer Guide to Healthcare and Wellness
    McGraw-Hill/Health Professions Division (800/634–3966)

NATIONAL HEALTHCARE MARKETING ASSOCIATIONS

The Alliance for Healthcare Strategy and Marketing (312/704–9700)
The American Marketing Association (800/262–1150)
The Society for Healthcare Strategy and Market Development (312/422–3888)

MISCELLANEOUS

Calendar of Health Observances & Recognition Days from the American Hospital Association (800/242–2626)
Catalog of public health publications, Sage Publications (805/499–9774)

Bibliography

THE FOLLOWING ARTICLES, publications, books, references, and web sites have all been used in researching and writing this book. The specific books listed will increase your understanding of healthcare dynamics, strategic marketing, sales management, the selling process, customer service, and self-improvement.

HEALTHCARE

A Short History of Medicine, E. H. Ackerknecht, Baltimore, MD: John Hopkins University Press, 1982

Health Care Consumers in the 1990s, R. K. Thomas, Ithaca, NY: American Demographic Books, 1992

Health Against Wealth, George Anders, Boston: Houghton Mifflin Co., 1996

Health and Healthcare in the United States, County and Metro Area Data, Lanham, MD: Bernan Press, 1999

Healthcare Finance for the Non-Finance Manager, Louis Gapenski, Chicago: Probus Publishing, 1994

Hospital Departmental Profiles, Chicago: American Hospital Publishing, Inc., 1990

Medical Sociology, William C. Cockerham, Upper Saddle River, NJ: Prentice-Hall, 1998

Medicine on Trial, Charles B. Inlander, Lowell S. Levin and Ed Weiner, New York: Prentice-Hall, 1988

Not What the Doctor Ordered, Jeffrey C. Bauer, New York: McGraw-Hill, 1998

Silent Violence, Silent Death: The Hidden Epidemic of Medical Malpractice, Harvey Rosenfield, Washington, DC: Essential Information, 1994

Statistical Abstract of the United States, U.S. Department of Commerce, Economics and Statistics Administration, Bureau of the Census, 1999.

The Best Medicine, Robert Arnot, M.D., Reading, MA: Addison-Wesley Publishing Co., 1992

The Great White Lie: How American's Hospitals Betray Our Trust and Endanger Our Lives, Walt Bogdanich, New York: Simon & Schuster, 1991

The Crisis in Healthcare: Costs, Choices, and Strategies, Dean C. Coddington, David J. Keen, Keith D. Moore, and Richard Clark, San Francisco: Jossey-Bass, Inc., 1990

The Health Care Book of Lists, Richard K. Thomas, Louis G. Pol, and William F. Sehnert, Jr., Winter Park, FL: GR Press, 1994

Working Together: Building Integrated Healthcare Organizations Through Improved Executive/Physician Collaboration, Seth Allcorn, Chicago: Probus Publishing, 1995

The American Way of Death–Revisited, Jessica Mitford, New York: Alfred A. Knopf Publisher, 1998

USING THE TELEPHONE

Cold Calling Techniques, Stephan Schiffman, Holbrook, MA: Adams Media Corp., 1999

Powerful Telephone Skills, Hawthorne, NJ: Career Press, 1993

FAX MARKETING

FAX This Book, John Caldwell, New York: Workman Publishing, 1990

BODY LANGUAGE

Body Language, Julius Fast, New York: MJF Books, 1970
Body Language, Gordon R. Wainwright, Lincolnwood, IL: NTC
  Publishing Group, 1993
Signals: How to Use Body Language for Power, Success, and Love,
  Allan Pease, New York: Bantam Books, 1984

MARKETING

Building the Strategic Plan, Stephanie K. Marrus, New York:
  John Wiley & Sons, 1984
Guerrilla Marketing, Jay Conrad Levinson, Boston: Houghton
  Mifflin Co., 1994
Guerrilla Advertising, Jay Conrad Levinson, Boston: Houghton
  Mifflin Co., 1994
Guerrilla P.R., Michael Levine, New York: Harper Business, 1993
Healthcare Advertising and Marketing: A Practical Approach, Pat
  Meade, New York: McGraw-Hill, 1999
Healthcare Market Research, Erik N. Berkowitz, Louis G. Pol,
  and Richard K. Thomas, Burr Ridge, IL: Irwin Publishing,
  1997
How to Write a Successful Marketing Plan, Roman G. Hiebing
  and Scott W. Cooper, Lincolnwood, IL: NTC Business
  Books, 1997
The Information Please Business Almanac and Desk Reference,
  Boston: Houghton Mifflin Co., 1999
Lesko's Info-Power, Matthew Lesko, Kensington, MD: Informa-
  tion USA, 1990
*AMA Handbook for Managing Business-to-Business Marketing
  Communications*, J. Nicholas De Bonis and Roger S. Peter-
  son, Lincolnwood, IL: NTC Business Books, 1997
Market Mapping, Sunny Baker and Kim Baker, New York:
  McGraw-Hill, 1993

Market Research Handbook for Healthcare Professionals, Paul H. Keckley, Chicago: American Hospital Publishing, Inc., 1988

Marketing For Healthcare Organizations, Philip Kotler and Roberta N. Clarke, Englewood Cliffs, NJ: Prentice Hall, 1987

Marketing Research, H. Robert Dodge, Sam Fullerton, and David Rink, Columbus, OH: Charles E. Merrill Publishing Company, 1982

Radiology Manager's Handbook, Eric A. Bouchard, Dubuque, IA: Sheperd, Inc., 1992

Marketing Myths That Are Killing Business, Kevin J. Clancy and Robert S. Shulman, New York: McGraw Hill, 1994

Business Planning Guide, David H. Bangs, Jr., Portsmouth, NH: Upstart Publishing Co., 1978

The Perfect Business Plan Made Simple, William Lasher, New York: Doubleday, 1994

The New Competitor Intelligence, Leonard M. Fuld, New York: John Wiley & Sons, Inc., 1995

The 22 Immutable Laws of Marketing, Al Ries and Jack Trout, New York: Harper Business, 1993

Getting the Most from Your Yellow Pages Advertising: Maximum Profits and Minimum Cost, Barry Maher, Middletown, RI: Aegis Publishing Group, 1997

PRESENTATIONS

Presentations Plus, David Peoples' Proven Techniques, New York: John Wiley & Sons, Inc., 1992

I Can See You Naked: A Fearless Guide to Making Great Presentations, Ron Hoff, Kansas City, MO: Andrews and McMeel, 1988

COMPETITIVE INTELLIGENCE

Competitive Intelligence for the Competitive Edge, Alan Dutka, Chicago: American Marketing Association, 1999.

NEGOTIATING

How to Negotiate Anything with Anyone Anywhere Around the World, Frank L. Acuff, New York: AMACOM, 1997

Negotiate Like the Pros, John Patrick Dolan, New York: Perigee Books, 1992

The Art of Negotiating, Gerard I. Nierenberg, New York: Simon and Schuster, 1986

The Negotiating Game, Chester L. Karrass, New York: Harper Business, 1992

Getting to Yes: Negotiating Agreement Without Giving In, Roger Davis and William Ury, New York: Penguin Books, 1991

Never Be Lied to Again, David J. Lieberman, New York: St. Martin's Press, 1998

How to Argue and Win Every Time, Gerry Spence, New York: St. Martin's Griffin, 1996

The Fast Forward MBA in Negotiating and Deal Making, Roy J. Lewicki and Alexander Hiam, New York: John Wiley & Sons, 1999

CUSTOMER SERVICE

Ultimate Patient Satisfaction, John O'Malley, New York: Mc-Graw-Hill, 1997

Kaizen, the Key to Japan's Competitive Success, Masaaki Imai, New York: Random House Business Division, 1986

The Customer Connection: Quality for the Rest of Us, John Guaspari, New York: AMACOM, 1998

How To Win Customers and Keep Them for Life, Michael LeBoeuf, New York: Putnam's Sons, 1987

Measuring and Managing Patient Satisfaction, William J. Krowinski and Steven R. Steiver, Chicago: American Hospital Publishing, Inc., 1996

Take This Book to the Hospital With You, Charles B. Inlander and Ed Weiner, Allentown, PA: People's Medical Society, 1997

Cultural Competence Compendium, Chicago: American Medical Association, 1995
The Survey Kit, Thousand Oaks, CA: Sage Publications, 1995

PERSONAL IMPROVEMENT

Eat Smart-Think Smart, Robert Haas, New York: Harper Collins, 1994
Jumping the Curve, Nicholas Imparato and Oren Harari, San Francisco: Jossey-Bass, Inc., 1994
Mentally Tough, Dr. James E. Loehr, New York: M. Evans and Company, Inc., 1996
The Memory Book, Lorayne & Lucas, Stein & Day

HEALTHCARE BOOKS AND ARTICLES BY JOHN O'MALLEY

Ultimate Patient Satisfaction: Tips, Tools, and Techniques for Achieving UPS, New York: McGraw-Hill, 1997
Managed Care Referral: How to Develop a Systematic Approach for Building Your Referral Business in Today's Healthcare Environment, Chicago: Irwin Professional Publishing, 1996
94 Strategies for Referral Development: A Guide to Growing your Diagnostic Imaging Business, San Francisco: Miller Freeman Inc., 1994
"Medigraphics: A New Perspective on Healthcare Markets," *AMA Marketing News* vol. 22, no. 10 (May 9, 1998)

HEALTHCARE-RELATED WEB SITES

Agency for Healthcare and Quality Research
   http://www.ahcpr.gov
American College of Healthcare Executives
   http://www.ache.org

American Chiropractic Association
  http://www.amerchiro.org
American Hospital Directory
  http://www.ahd.com
American Medical Association
  http://www.ama-assn.org
Association for Death Education and Counseling
  http://www.adec.org
CAPWEB: The Internet Guide to the United States Congress
  http://www.capweb.net
Centers for Disease Control and Prevention
  http://www.cdc.gov
Columbia University Health Service
  http://www.cc.columbia.edu/cu/health/
County and City Data Book (U.S. Census Bureau)
  http://www.census.gov/statab/www/ccdb.html
Dartmouth Atlas of Healthcare in the United States
  http://www.dartmouthatlas.org
Dr. Koop
  http://www.drkoop.com
EthnoMed: Ethnic Medicine Guide
  http://www.hslib.washington.edu/clinical/ethnomed/
  index.html
Federal Government/Benchmarking Consortium Study Report
  http://www.npr.gov/library/papers/benchmrk/bstprac.html
Florida Hospitals Discharge Data
  http://www.hbsi.com
HCPUnet: Hospital Ratings
  http://www.ahrq.gov/data/hcup/hcupnet.htm
Healthfinder: Federal Government Healthcare Database
  http://www.healthfinder.gov
HealthGrades: The Healthcare Rating Experts
  http://www.healthgrades.com

Health and Literacy Compendium
   http://hub1.worlded.org/health/comp/index.html
*Department of Health and Human Services Office of the Inspector
   General*
   www.oig.gov
Last Acts: Care and Caring at the End of Life
   http://www.lastacts.org
MayoClinic Health Oasis
   http://www.mayohealth.org
Med Help
   http://www.medhlp.netusa.net/index.html
MRN: Medical Products and Equipment
   http://www.mrn.com
Medical Headlines
   http://www.ivanhoe.com
Medical Matrix
   http://www.medmatrix.org
MedicineNet
   http://www.medicinenet.com
Medline (National Library of Medicine)
   http://www.nlm.nih.gov
Medsite: Health & Medical Information
   http://www.medsite.com
Merck Manual of Diagnosis & Therapy
   http://www.merck.com/pubs/mmanual
National Center for Complementary Medicine
   http://www.altmed.od.nih.gov
National Center for Health Statistics
   http://www.cdc.gov/nchs
National Committee for Quality Assurance
   http://www.ncqa.org
National Health Information Center
   http://www.cmhc.com

National Institutes of Health
    http://www.nih.gov
National Library of Medicine
    http://www.nlm.nih.gov
Nursing/Medical Humor on the Internet
    http://www.wwnurse.com/nursing/humor
On Health
    http://www.onhealth.com
PubMed (search service)
    http://www.ncbi.nlm.nih.gov/pubmed
RxList: The Internet Drug Index
    http://www.rxlist.com
Supportive Care of the Dying
    http://www.careofdying.org
Surgeon General
    http://www.surgeongeneral.gov
Statistical Universe (Congressional Information Service, Inc.)
    http://www.cispubs.com
U.S. Census Bureau
    http://.www.census.gov
U.S. General Accounting Office
    http://www.ssdc.ucsd.edu/gpo/gao.html
U.S. Department of Justice
    http://www.usdoj.gov
U.S. Bureau of Labor Statistics
    http://www.bls.gov
U.S. Department of Transportation, Bureau of Transportation Statistics
    http://www.bts.gov
WebMD
    http://my.wcbmd.com

About the Author

JOHN F. O'MALLEY IS a nationally recognized author, consultant, and speaker with more than 25 diversified years in corporate senior management planning, marketing, and sales positions within the healthcare industry. Mr. O'Malley specializes in business development, customer/patient satisfaction, and sales, and is president and founder of Strategic Visions Inc, a Birmingham, Alabama–based company that provides impact thinking, positioning, planning services, and sales and service training.

Mr. O'Malley's marketing and advertising efforts have won many awards, including the Bronze Quill, the Golden Star, and the 11th Annual Healthcare Advertising Awards, brochure category Gold and overall Best of Show. He is also the founder and sponsor of National Patient Recognition Week and Day, recognized by the American Society for Healthcare Marketing and Public Relations as the first week of February and February 3rd, respectively. He has appeared on radio talk shows and has had articles in the following national publications: the American Marketing Association's *Marketing News*, the *Journal of Healthcare Marketing*, *Hospital and Health Networks*, the *Alliance for Healthcare Strategy and Marketing*, *Diagnostic Imaging*, *M.D. News*, *Selling Power*, and *USA Today*.

This is the author's fourth healthcare book. His others include *Ninety-Four Referral Development Strategies for Imaging Centers* (Miller Freeman Publishing 1994); *Managed Care Referral* (Irwin Professional Publishing 1996); and *Ultimate Patient Satisfaction* (McGraw-Hill 1997).